REFLECTIONS FOR A CAREGIVER

JO KEMP

Mary Ann & Toni:
Be blessed in
all you do

Warmly
Jo Kemp

ISBN: 1-4196-9539-8

ISBN-13: 9781419695391

Visit www.booksurge.com to order additional copies.

TO MY HUSBAND BOB
My best friend and the light of my life

INTRODUCTION

After working with thousands of caregivers, I realized there was an overwhelming need for daily support and encouragement. I have a passion for all caregivers but especially for those who care for a person with Alzheimer's or a related dementia. Working with caregivers and being a caregiver has given me insight as to what caregivers needs really are. I know that some days are a struggle and they do not know if they can go on. Caregivers often feel alone and are consumed in their caregiver role.

More than anything I want caregivers to know: "you are doing a great job; it's more than ok to take care of yourself first, asking for help is the right thing to do, you have nothing to feel guilty about, you have the right to take pride in what you do, and to know that the decisions you make are in the best interest of your loved one." It is my hope that this book gives them the courage to reach out.

The wisdom is not all mine, but that of the many caregivers that shared their journey with me. They have shared with me some of their deepest thoughts and feelings. It is my hope that through this daily read book you can find knowledge and peace of mind. You can use each days read as a guide to problem solving or as a vehicle for reflections. Working for the Alzheimer's Association for seven years gave me the opportunity to follow my passion of helping caregivers. I believe that caregivers should receive all the physical, emotional, and spiritual help available. This book addresses a topic in a short form and at the same time empowers caregivers to keep up their good work.

In reference to the person you are caring for; the words loved one is used. The mention of God refers to the highest power as he affects your life.

Although this book has been written for family caregivers, it is my hope that every facility, adult day care, hospital or any place that cares for Alzheimer's patients, will keep copies handy for their staff to read. Professional caregivers experience many of the same feelings and fears that family caregivers do.

Maya Angelou says, "The idea is to write it so that people hear it and it slides through the brain to the heart" It is my hope that this book will do just that.

January

What great thing would you attempt
if you knew you could not fail?

DR. ROBERT H. SCHULLER

New Year

A new year's resolution is usually a commitment to change something in our life that causes us difficulty. The problem with making resolutions is that we do it with unrealistic expectations. We cannot stop smoking, drinking and go on a diet all at the same time. Studies show that people who make impulsive resolutions are less likely to stick to them. Maybe a better approach to our new year is to make a list of things we would like to accomplish in the next 12 months. It could be as simple as cleaning out the junk drawer that has been driving us crazy. Believe it or not there is a lot of satisfaction from such simple acts. We might also want to include fun things such as taking a vacation alone. Sound impossible but it's not. Simple steps can bring big results.

*I will approach the New Year
with realistic expectations of myself.*

Perfection

There is no glory in being a perfectionist. It will not win us more love, acceptance, or fulfillment. By striving to be a perfectionist, we will set our standards too high and beyond reason. Trying to obtain these high standards, we become preoccupied and set ourselves up for failure. The fear of failure and self-disapproval can be overwhelming. It is far better to strive to do our very best. Our standards will still be high, but obtainable. In the perfectionist's world, there is a right way and a wrong way. There is no middle ground. This mindset truly is unrealistic. We need to see our mistakes as opportunities for growth and learning. More importantly, we need to give ourselves credit for what we do well, even if it is not perfect.

I will try not to be perfect, but I will be the best I can.

Sands of the Past Hour Glass

Early on in the disease, our loved one will lose their sense of time, because they cannot reason they have no way to measure the passage of time. Right after they have finished a meal they may ask to eat again. Nights and days become confused and they may get restless and begin to wander around the house and yes they may want to eat again. Their lives become the past. They may think they need to get home to their mothers and they are worried about being late. They can become uncooperative when we want them to fit into our time schedule. If we take things slow and easy, we will have a better chance of accomplishing things that need to be done. There life will soon become an hour-glass that is only filed with the sands of the past.

I will slow down my pace, enjoy the present,
and not try to make my loved one fit into my timetable.

Self Pity

Self-pity is a form of self-indulgence. It blocks reality and lets in negative thoughts. If we continue to doubt ourselves, it could lead to self- pity. If we throw a "pity party" for ourselves, we can be assured that no one will come. We need to change our focus from what we cannot do, to what we can do. By changing our focus and making it more positive, we allow ourselves the opportunity to see things as they really are. We are the only ones that can change this self-indulgent pattern. Life can be very hard when we are mired in self-pity. It is also difficult to make informed decisions when we are filled with self-pity. Eliminating self-pity will allow our lives to flow more smoothly and we will feel less stressed. A glass half empty is hardly worth taking a drink.

Today I will examine my life focus
so that my glass is always half full.

$\mathcal{D}enial$

When this disease started, we were in denial or maybe we just did not know what it was. We may have thought it was just old age. We thought that old age breeds memory loss. We cannot continue to stay in denial after the diagnosis is given, because we will end up defeating ourselves. We cannot afford to continue this pattern because there is much planning to be done. We need to find out about resources that are available to us. Financial and health care decisions need to be made. Safety issues in our home need to be addressed. We also need to make plans for our loved one in case of emergency. If we continue to deny we are disowning responsibilities, we will soon lose control over important issues. By putting our denial in the past we can now begin to move forward.

It does not matter if I have been in denial in the past for today I will take ownership and regain control

Accidents Happen

Accidents happen and sometimes they happen in the middle of our living room floor. Although this may be disturbing to us, we must not react to the situation. No one would relieve themselves inappropriately on purpose. Our caregiving journey will be filled with these unexpected moments. If we learn to cope with things early on in the disease, it will be much easier as the disease progresses. We have the power to control our reactions and this is the time to take that control, so that we do not over react. Everything our loved one does should be considered failure free. Yes, even relieving themselves in the plant in the living room. It is difficult to treat these types of problems with calm and sensitivity, but our well-being as well as theirs will be at stake.

I will be sensitive to my loved one's behavior,
and do what I can to make their environment failure free.

Walking

We take for granted the ability to walk and be independent. Most people have been doing it since they took those first steps as an infant. As our loved one's disease progress, they may encounter problems with walking. They may also have a problem with negotiating turns or keeping their balance. The most frightening thing about these events is that they cannot comprehend that there is a problem, and no amount of reminding them will change their actions. They will try to stand up and walk even though they cannot, because the brain just has not gotten the message. Our job now is to evaluate possible risks in our homes and modify them as best we can for their safety. It is a lot better to take precautionary measures rather than waiting for an accident to happen.

I will evaluate the safety of my home
and monitor my loved one's walking ability.

Forgiveness

Forgiveness is often viewed as a weakness. It is just the opposite. In order to forgive we must be strong. Forgiveness is powerful. Forgiveness does not mean we minimize or deny what a person has done, but it does mean that we should not be judgmental or resentful of them. In reality, we are not forgiving the person, but what the person has done. Forgiveness is not about someone else, it is about us. Forgiving others and ourselves is one of the greatest gifts we have. When we choose to forgive, we open the doors of the present and future, and give ourselves the gift of today. To quote Mahatma Gandhi; "The weak can never forgive. Forgiveness is the attribute of the strong. Forgiveness is the inner strength that helps us heal and liberates our soul."

*Today I will release the past, and forgive myself
so that I can be ready for the future.*

Who are you?

Today, my loved one thought I was their mother, sister, or just the nice person who comes to visit. For a moment, I thought my heart would break, and I felt the pain of losing one more part of their existence. Even though we knew this day might come, we are never prepared for the flood of feelings and emotions that it evokes. For a moment, we felt rejected and unloved. We know these feelings are not valid and that they do love us they just do not recognize us at this moment. It is so difficult at times like this not to show our fear and sorrow. We know that no matter how hard it is we need to rise above the occasion. The kindest gift we can give to them and ourselves is one of soft loving reassurance that we will always be there for them.

Even though my loved one does not recognize me,
I will reassure them that I will always be there for them

Burdens

We can place tremendous burdens on ourselves. We can be our own worst enemy. We believe that we need to get everything done today and we should do it faster and better. We literally sabotage ourselves before we even get started. We waste a tremendous amount of energy when we place ourselves in this negative mode. So what is the worst thing that can happen if we do not accomplish all we want to do today? Are the caregiver police going to arrest us? It is difficult to accomplish things when we feel burdened. The more pressure we place upon ourselves the less likely we are to succeed. We do not need to prove anything to others. We do not have to answer to anyone but our higher power. We need to accept who we are, and remember that we are doing the best we can, and that is enough.

I will stop looking at things as burdens but rather as blessings.

Feeling and Emotions

It is ok to express our feelings, its part of taking care of ourselves. It is valid to express our feeling as long as we do not hurt others. Sometimes we find it difficult to express them because things we heard as a child have programmed us: boys do not cry, do not trust your feelings, or keep a stiff upper lip. We have internalized these messages and they lead us into negative self-talk. We need to feel what we feel, and at times cry if we need to cry. By reprogramming these childhood messages, we allow ourselves to have control over when and how we will express them. If we do not express our feelings, others will not know where we stand or what our needs are. Our feelings and emotions can be very therapeutic when we know how to use them constructively.

I will us my feelings in a constructive manner
and take control over my emotions.

January 12

Compassionate Communication

When we speak to a child, we do so with compassion. We do not argue with them because it is not an option. People that have dementia do not always get this type of compassion. Their minds are slowing down and they are losing the ability to reason, yet we speak harshly to them and argue, as if they could understand and correct their behavior. Whatever our pattern of communication was with them in the past, it will no longer work, especially as they progress in the disease. We now need to use simple sentences and cues to help them understand what we are saying. We should listen carefully to what they say and be aware of their body language. The more we comprehend, the better our communication will be. Compassionate communication should be something we extend to all people, but especially to our loved one.

I will strive for better communication skills
so that I may understand and appreciate my loved one's needs

Unconditional love

As caregivers, we must have unconditional love for the person we care for. Caring for those with Alzheimer's and related dementias is love without limitation or conditions. We have to accept them for who they are and where they are in their life now. We cannot change their behavior when this disease takes over their mind and body, no matter how trying the behavior may be. An approach of reward or punishment will not work. Using the "whatever works" approach will allow us to love unconditionally. We also need to have this love for ourselves, and treat ourselves with the gentle kindness we give to our loved one. Being a caregiver allows us the greatest opportunity to give and receive unconditional love.

Today I will treat myself and my loved one
with unconditional love

January 14

Personal Inventory

Occasionally we become so focused on what we don't have that we do not recognize what we do have. We dream of having the perfect home, the perfect family, and the riches that should be ours after our many years of working and raising a family. Many of these riches are right in front of us, but we cannot see them because we are only looking at what we think we do not have. If we take time to do a quiet personal inventory, we will find that our home is quite adequate, our families are doing well, and we have the money we need to care for our loved one and ourselves. If there is a gap in our relationship with our family or friends, then there is no time like the present to take steps to fix it. Our family and friends can be the wealth of our existence if we open our hearts and let them in.

I will look for all I do have in my life
and not dwell on what I do not have.

Don't Miss It

If we are not careful, we could miss it; the twinkle in their eye that says, "I'm happy", the soft smile that says "thank you" or the sigh of comfort that says, "I feel safe when you are with me." These are just a few of the links in the chain of love that our loved one gives to us. Their expressions are like spoken words that let us know how much they love and appreciate us. If they could speak the words, they would let us know that we make a difference in their life. We have a special bond with our loved one and these special moments go a long way in helping us through our day. They put the joy in caring. They are a testament of unspoken appreciation and they are there for us to see if we take the time to recognize them.

I will watch for the unspoken gestures of love
that my loved offers up to me and be glad for them.

Be True to Yourself

Sometimes it is hard to be true to ourselves. We let other people's thinking influence how we feel. Good old Dr Suess pegs it, "Be who you are and say what you feel, because those who mind don't matter, and those who matter don't mind". The fact of the matter is that most people do not care. They have their own problems. We are unique individuals and we need to trust our instincts. Using our mental toughness and not giving up when the going gets tough is a testament to our wholeness. Gloom and doom have no place in our life. If we cannot be true to ourselves, we certainly cannot be true to others. Our self worth is not dependent on what others think. In the end, the most important thing is to be ourselves and be our own best friend.

I will be my own best friend and trust in myself.

Realistic Expectations

Keeping our expectations at a reasonable level allows us to perform our daily activities with out self recrimination. We are doing more things for our loved one as their disease progresses. As our tasks increase, so does our stress level. We try to be all things to all people. As our work increases we begin to wonder why we feel so tired and why every thing seems so monumental. Our common sense tells us it is impossible to be all things to all people, and yet we continue to knock ourselves out trying. This is the time we need to stop, step back, and evaluate our situation and be realistic about what we can and can not do. We all have our limitations we just need to recognize them, move on, and ask for the help if needed. We are caregivers not magicians.

Being kind to ourselves
is the kindest thing we can do for our loved one.

Generosity

Being generous is an admirable trait, but sometimes we as caregivers are generous to a fault. We do not know how to say no. Even when we are at our wit's end, we want to please, thus we give in to various requests from our family and friends. We go places we do not want to go. We do things we really do not want to do. Saying that we do this because we are too tired to argue about it is no excuse. Although it is sometimes difficult to tell someone no, in the end we will feel relieved, and some of the daily pressure will be lessened. Family traditions and requests can be modified to suit our needs. No one said it was easy, but it is necessary, and we do not have to feel guilty about it. Generosity is noble, but when it jeopardizes our well-being or that of our loved one, it does not hold this quality.

Today I will take a stand and politely say no
to request that are overwhelming to my loved one or me.

Dreams

No matter how desperate our lives may feel at times, there is always room to dream. Dreams can be magical and can give us the strength to move forward. They are the light at the end of the tunnel. We do not have to give up our dreams because we are now caregivers. As hard as it is to think about it, there is life after caregiving. We have many demands on our lives, our dreams may have been buried, but now it is time to revive them. When we reconnect to them, they will give us hope. We may not be able to fulfill them as soon as we would like, but we still will be able to realize them. We do not need to change our dreams. We just need to change the timing of them. Dreams give us something to look forward to. They make us happy and happiness makes us healthy.

I will rediscover my dreams and take joy in them.

Understand

Someone may says thing to us such as, "don't worry they don't understand anyways". Such statements can make us angry at their ignorance. They have just crossed the dignity line. We really do not know how much our loved one understands, but talking about them in this manner is unacceptable. This is a time when we really need to step back, take a deep breath and regroup our thoughts. If possible we need to take the person aside and explain to them what we know about the disease, and how we feel about their remark. We do not need to be nasty because truly they may not have known that what they said was cruel and inappropriate. People who do not live with this disease have no real understanding of the depth of hurt and anguish we go through daily as our loved one slowly slips away.

I will strive to make people understand this disease
so that they do not cross the dignity line with my loved one.

Looking for the Clues

Part of our caregiver life is being a good detective. This will be even more important as the disease progress and their communication skills decline. Opportunities for problem solving are with us every day. Sometimes we do not know what our loved one wants, but by careful listening and observation we may find a clue to their needs. Because of the deep cognitive decline that propels this disease, we become the sole detective and problem solver. We also need to learn to anticipate their needs by observing how they act or react at certain times of the day. Even when we do not totally understand their needs, our mere presence, and unconditional love will comfort and help them feel safe.

I will look at problem solving
as an opportunity to meet the needs of my loved one

Peace of Mind

Our happiness is one component that contributes to our emotional health and health of our body. It is a feeling we get from knowing we are safe and our needs are being met. There are times when we must change our expectations to attain happiness and peace of mind. If we dwell on our unhappiness, peace of mind will escape us. Like dignity, we sometimes do not recognize happiness until we do not have it. Like all good things, being at peace is a process that needs to be worked on in order to be attained. We can begin by accept what cannot be changed. This will save a lot of time and energy. We can also practice being more patient and tolerant with people. Abraham Lincoln once said, "Most folks are about as happy as they make up their minds to be."

I will strive for peace of mind
so that I can be happy in my life.

Comfort Zone

If our actions do not serve our best interest, then why do we hold onto them? Sometimes it is easier not to change how we think or feel because in order to do so, we must step out of our comfort zone. We have put a lot of work into ensuring that certain things in our lives remain constant. We have conditioned ourselves in such a manner that we have put up mental boundaries that keep us from moving forward. In order to grow and try new things, we need to take the first step outside our comfort zone. Stepping out of this zone will allow us to learn new things and feel more confident in our abilities. It is easier to expand our comfort zone in small, steady, steps rather than in great big leaps. Just because we have "always done it that way" does not make it the best way.

I will step out of my comfort zone
so that I can move forward and learn new things.

Little Things

Life really is not about the big things. It is the little things that count. Holding a hand when they are afraid, quietly listening when they struggle with their thoughts or saying I love you, these are the little things when strung together makes them big. They could be considered little acts of kindness that take very little time or energy. These spontaneous actions can make such a difference in a person's quality of life. Little things in life are so important that many love songs have been written about them. "Blow me a kiss from across the room; say I look nice when I'm not. Send me the warmth of a secret smile to show me you have not forgot. For always and ever, now and forever little things mean a lot." Who doesn't remember this song by Kitty Kallen in 1962? It kindled many hearts to fall in love and do little thing out of love.

*I will value the little things in life
and remember that little things mean a lot.*

Hopelessness

Hopelessness is a kin to helplessness. Hopelessness is such an empty feeling, and it eventually makes us the victim of negative reasoning. Our lives as caregivers may not be the vision of completeness, but we should never give up hope. When we feel hopeless, we miss so much in our life. The small good things begin to be covered by the negativity. Our negativity becomes so powerful that it is difficult for us to see the positives in our life. It blocks us from finding solutions to our problems. Because we feel helpless we stop taking positive actions, and negative things begin to happen. If we replace hopelessness with hope, we may be disappointed at times, but we will learn to overcome obstacles resulting in positive solutions to our problems.

I will hold onto hope even in the face of adversity

Compassion

Compassion should not be reserved just for other people. It is not something that is there for us to give away. It is important to be compassionate with ourselves. This is not a selfish act. It is a positive way to keep in touch with our own feelings. When we use self- talk, we are usually responding to fear or guilt. We tend to beat ourselves up when things go badly. Having compassion for ourselves means that we honor and accept our humanness. We will also make mistakes or bad choices, but that does not make us a bad or unworthy person. It is just part of our human life experiences. Self-compassion allows us to treat ourselves kindly, and lay aside our self-guilt. It helps us maintain our own balance. Self-compassion lets us treat ourselves with the same kindness we would show a friend in need.

I will treat myself with the same compassion I show others.

Anger

We all feel anger throughout our lives. Anger is not the enemy; it is what we do with the anger that can make it so. Anger has different levels, from just being upset to full-blown rage. Anger is a call to action. It is an emotion that left unattended can lead to mistreatment of the one we care for. It heightens our negative feelings towards others and ourselves. Suppressed anger only leads to roadblocks that are difficult to overcome. We are the only ones that can control our anger and we need to control our anger before it controls us. We also need to control our outward behavior, as well as our internal response to the anger. Mitch Albom in the book *The Five People You Meet in Heaven* says," Holding anger is a poison, it eats you from the inside".

Today I will acknowledge my anger
and work on using it for positive action in my daily life

Day Care

"I could never put my loved one in day care" "The people there are much worse than he is" "He wouldn't go even if I asked him to" "They wouldn't know how to care for him". These are just a few of the excuse we have when confronted with the possibility of having our loved one attend day care. Instead of thinking about its advantages, out of fear, we only see the negative side. Day care lets our loved one interact socially with peers, and share in stimulating activities while being cared for in a safe environment. Studies have shown that it can deter premature placement in residential care. Adult day care is a win-win solution. Recognizing that this is a big step for our loved one, and us we need to give the program a reasonable time for adjustment. Believe it or not, our loved one will probably adjust better to the change then we do.

I will stop making excuses
and explore the option of day care for my loved one.

Tears

From the time we were very little, we were told not to cry. Somehow we have become convinced that it is wrong to cry. So now, we view crying as a sign of weakness and fear letting the tears flow. We may be told to "just deal with it". The thought of crying when others are around makes us feel vulnerable. Washington Irving said, "There is sacredness in tears. They are not the mark of weakness, but the power. They speak more eloquently than ten thousand tongues. They are the messengers of overwhelming grief and the unspeakable love". We should not keep our tear bottled up inside. This does not mean we should bawl every time something goes wrong. Everything in moderation, but crying from time to time can be cathartic; it can be good for the soul as well as the body. It also said that, "tears are the safety valve of our mind's heart".

I will use my tears to cleanse my heart and soul.

Aha Moments

An "Aha." moment is one of those times in our life where all the pieces fall into place. It is when we have found the last piece of the puzzle, and can now see the whole picture. Basically it's when something happens in our life that makes us stand up and take notice and think, so that's what it's all about, or that's the answer. It is also referred to as a light bulb moment or an epiphany. No matter what they are called, they are a welcome solution to a problem. They usually happen when we are in a relaxed state of mind, and have set the problem aside. When we are frustrated, anxious, or fixated on a problem the solution rarely comes to us. We can not create these moments. In fact, the more we try the harder it gets. These are defining moments when what we have been working on or thinking about becomes crystal clear. Because these moments tend to come in times of clarity, it is even more important that we take time for ourselves to rest our bodies and minds.

*I will use my quiet times
to clarify my mind and rest my body.*

Meditation

Meditation is a type of self-care activity that all caregivers should at least try. There is no right or wrong behavior during meditation. We all have the ability to consciously relax. Because our minds are filled with everyday clutter, random thoughts will creep into our mind as we begin to meditate, and that is ok, it is normal. What we need to do first is focus on our breathing. Even though this may be difficult in the beginning, it can be done. We should not become discouraged if the thoughts show up in flashes or we hear other noises. The more we try to meditate, the better we will get. The hardest thing is not to get discouraged. If we can meditate for even ten minutes, we will be clearer of mind and relaxed in spirit. The following is a good description on learning to meditate: Meditation is very much like training a puppy. You put the puppy down and say, "Stay" Does the puppy listen? It gets up and it runs away. You sit the puppy back down again. "Stay." And the puppy runs away over and over again. Sometimes the puppy jumps up, runs over, and pees in the corner or makes some other mess. Our minds are much the same as the puppy, only they create even bigger messes. In training the mind, or the puppy, we have to start over and over again. From *A Path with Heart"*

I will practice meditation
so that I may be more relaxed and focused.

February

Anyone can give up; it's the easiest thing in the world to do. However, to hold it together when everyone else would understand if you fell apart, that is true strength.

UNKNOWN

Issues

We've heard the term "End of Life Issues". It's too bad that our life's end has to be an issue. Everyone wants to have a peaceful, pain-free death, but the failure to make our needs known and put in writing is what precipitates the issue. It's not enough to just talk about them and promise to carry them out. In most cases, if it is not in writing, it is not going to happen. We take great care in planning how we want to live, but when it comes to what we want done when we are dying, we ignore it or procrastinate and do not have a plan. Even if it is too late for our loved one to write out their advance directives and living will, it is not too late for us. Like life, we only have one death; may it be dignified, painless, and filled with no regrets.

I will take control of my end of life decisions and not make them an issue that others will be burdened with.

Role Changes

Dealing with role changes is one of the hardest things we will have to deal with. Our spouse may not be the person we married in body, or our parent is no longer the parental figure and life as we know it changes. As our loved ones changes, so does our relationship. For a spouse there are also changes in emotional and physical intimacy that were once shared. Because we have to take on so many responsibilities and make such important decisions it can become overwhelming. There is good news-there are some things that usually do not change, and that is their need for physical contact. By continuing to give hugs and reassuring pats we can help them and ourselves feel better. We need to remember the core of who they are is still there. We cannot renegotiate our roles but we can accept them with honor.

I will accept my role with honor and always treat my loved one with the dignity they deserve.

Feeling Good

Having dementia does not make our loved one any less unique or valued as a human being. They need to feel respect and value as much as anyone else does. It is up to us to help them feel good about themselves. We are the key person in their life, and we set the pace. Giving them failure-free tasks, or activities that fit their abilities, will give them a sense of achievement. Doing things with them rather than for them will help to keep them independent. It does not really matter that it takes them twice as long. Now we need to let them set their pace. It is not always easy to watch them struggle with a problem. We will know when to intervene. By being sensitive to their struggle we make it ok, no matter how it is done. Helping them feel good about themselves is a true expression of our love.

I will help my loved one feel good about themselves and keep them as independent as possible.

Superman or Woman

How do you eat an elephant? One bite at a time. This is also a good way to approach our daily tasks. By breaking them down into small steps and taking them one at a time, they become more manageable. Because we sometimes feel pressure to perform, we take on more that we can handle comfortably. We take on the superman persona. We think we can do anything single-handedly. The easier we make the task, the more apt it is to be done. If it takes a week to wash the windows, then so be it. What is the big rush anyways? If things begin to pile up, then it may be time to ask for help or to hire someone. We're good, but we aren't superman or woman. The most famous line in the Tao Te Ching, A written Chinese book of philosophy says it all; "A journey of a thousand miles begins with a single step."

I will take my tasks one-step at a time. If it is
not done today, so be it.

Mistakes and Opportunity

It is said that Thomas Edison failed 10,000 times before he perfected the light bulb. When asked how he felt about his 10,000 failures, he stated that he did not fail, but had learned 10,000 things that did not work. Maybe there is a positive side to making a mistake. If we stop looking at mistakes as bad, we will have the opportunity to learn from them. Every time we make a mistake, we get one-step closer to the solution. Mistakes are unintentional things we do wrong, but when used as a tool for learning, we make it right. We should not deny our mistakes because we cannot learn from something we do not acknowledge. Our mistakes become the opportunities and intentional lessons of life. There is an old axiom that goes; "If you're not making mistakes, you are not trying hard enough".

*I will look at my mistakes as opportunities to
learn and get it right.*

February 6

Losses

As our loved one begins to have physical and mental losses, we may begin to be consumed by our losses. Each time they lose a function or ability we begin to grieve. Because this disease is plagued by losses, we find it difficult to focus on their positive moments. By focusing only on these losses, we will lose the positive moments and the opportunity for positive interaction. Looking at what they can still do now and not projecting future losses, we can enjoy and hold these precious moments. As our loved one moves further into this disease, the special moments may be all we have left. It is all right to grieve these losses, but we must remember to celebrate even the smallest of positive moments. Living for today and rejoicing in the now will help us and our loved one to have more positive moments together.

Today I will rejoice in the abilities my loved one still has at this moment.

Support Groups

I do not want to go to a support group just to sit and listen to other people's problems. I have enough of my own. I do not have the time, and I certainly cannot leave them alone. All excuses aside, we really need to try them. As caregivers of loved ones with Alzheimer's disease, we need a place to come together and support each other through the sharing of our knowledge and experiences. Not all support groups are for everyone. By shopping around, we can find the one that suits our needs best. The key is to go a few times before we judge. Once we find a group we feel fits our needs, we should make it part of our survival routine. It is comforting to be able to share with people that are nonjudgmental and are taking the same journey we are.

I will look for a support group that I will feel comfortable attending and make it part of my survival plan.

Asking God

We have all heard the phrase "be careful what you ask for." Our loved ones constant repeating or asking of questions may be annoying to us, so we ask God to intervene and help them stop this behavior. If the behavior does not stop, we feel that God does not hear us or care about us. As irritating, as this behavior is there will come a time, when they will not be capable of doing even that, and we do not want to look back with regret. If we look back over our lives there were many time we did not get what we asked for. At the time, we may have been upset that our prayers were not answered but in the end, it was a good thing they were not. Our lives are constantly changing and we cannot dictate how we want everything to go. Our vision may be tunneled, but Gods is not.

I will trust that God know when and
how to answer my prayers.

We are Adults Now

The functionality or disfunctionality of our family's history often dictates if we chose to have them be part of our loved one's care. Before we set our plans into action we should try and reevaluate our family dynamics. First we need to remember that our past does not dictate our future. There may have been sibling rivalry that divided us and left business unfinished. Substance abuse or physical abuse may have been in our history. What-ever the problems were, we will be able to better serve our loved one if we come to terms with these issues. We are all grown up now and we need to act as the caring adults that we are. Setting aside our differences may allow us to work together. Working as a team is best when it is done out of love and respect for our loved one.

Out of love and respect for my loved one I will act as an adult, and strive to work as a team with my family.

Whisper

God's answer to our prayers will not come in a booming voice or as lightning from above. We may not even realize that our prayer has been answered, because the answer is not in the form we expected. God is under no obligation to answer yes to all our prayers. This may be a good thing since what we ask for is not always best for us. We also should not bargain with God. The "I will do this, if you will do that" approach will not work. God does not negotiate. We need to remember who is in charge, and that His timetable is not the same as ours. To pray for patience, and ask for it <u>right now</u> is a contradiction in itself. Be patient, the answer will come when we least expect it. He will softly place the answer in our mind and hearts.

I will stop negotiating with God and
patiently wait for His answers.

P_{ower}

There are times when we put ourselves down and give away our power. We down play our accomplishments. We let our vision of ourselves be tainted with doubt. We say yes when we mean no, and every time we agree when we do not, we give away power. We have been conditioned in childhood not to make waves and to do what we are told without question. We want to keep the peace no matter what, even if it is at our expense. The more we give away our power, the less we trust in ourselves. Our personal power comes from within. We know who we are and what we are capable of. When we give away our power and become passive, we have temporary won the battle but lost the war. There is no need to defer our power to others. By holding onto our power, we are able to make informed and affirmative decisions.

I will make informed decisions and not
give up my power to anyone.

February 12

Positive Emotions

We control our emotions. Our state of mind takes its lead from how we react to our emotions. It is impossible to be in a positive state of mind all the time, but if we are in a bad mood, nothing will seem right. Our problems will seem bigger, and we will lose perspective of the whole picture. Emotions have a purpose. The purpose of negative emotions is to help us survive and that of positive emotions to help us thrive. Changing how we feel is done in baby steps and with great thought. By changing our negative thoughts into positive ones, we take the first step towards contentment. Positive emotions will help us affirm the goodness in ourselves. We will be the person we want to be and the person that others want to be with.

I will affirm my positive thoughts, and move towards contentment for the betterment of my life.

Isolation

As our caregiving duties increase and our loved one's ability and mental capacity decreases, we tend to become socially isolated. Our daily lives begin to revolve exclusively around the needs of our loved one. Being isolated will eventually make us the next victim. Sometimes it just seems easier to avoid going out or asking others for assistance. To take ourselves out of isolation we must empower ourselves, ask for what we need, and be specific. We need to reconnect with our families and friends before we become so stressed that we lose focus on the world outside of caregiving. We need to understand that we are not alone and that it is ok to take a break and ask for help. We are naturally social creatures, and we need to stay that way.

Today I will speak up and share how I feel as I reconnect socially with my family and friends.

Love Today

There is a Buddhist quote that says, "You yourself, as much as anybody in the entire universe, deserve your love and affection." Even though we know this is true, we sometimes have a hard time doing it. So how do we start loving ourselves? We will begin by first saying nothing but good things about ourselves. We will throw caution to the wind and do something unexpected and special just for us. It could be dressing in our Hawaiian shirt and putting on some Hawaiian music, but what ever it is, it needs to be strictly for our pleasure. We can bask in our accomplishments and celebrate us. When we love ourselves, we are giving a big boost to our self-esteem. We are priceless human beings; there is no one else like us, and we deserve to be loved.

I am a priceless human being and I will love myself because I am worthy of it.

Creativeness

We do not have to be an artist or musician to be creative. The tender way we care for our loved one is creative. When we set goals and put a plan into action, we are being creative. Our creativity guides us to inspirational thoughts in times of stress. It lets us see all sides of a problem before we solve it. Creativity is merely a mental process wherein we generate new ideas and solutions to problems. Creativity is self-expression at its best. Sometimes creativity is about putting together ideas that do not seem to fit together naturally. Because of the progressive nature of Alzheimer's our approaches to their care is ever changing. We adjust to different events as they happen, or we learn to roll with the punches. Change is a catalyst for creativity and new ideas. As caregivers, we must learn to be flexible and work smarter.

I will use my creativity to enhance my care for my loved one.

Self-Acceptance

Self-acceptance is coming to an agreement with ourselves that we are not perfect, but we are doing the best we can in any particular moment in time. Looking back and thinking how we could have or should have done something different is setting us up for self-defeat. Our confidence in ourselves will be shaken. We should not ruminate on the "what ifs" of life. We need to focus on what we have learned from our experiences and apply them to our every day living. We do not have to measure up to other people's expectations. We are emotionally grounded and accept who we are, faults and all. When we have self-acceptance, we have a presence about us that leads others to take notice and they will want to be around us. If we do not believe in ourselves, we cannot expect others to believe in us either.

I will accept my self for who I am and have
confidence in what I do.

Courage

Maya Angelou has said, "One isn't necessarily born with courage, but one is born with potential". Courage is the ability to confront fear, pain, and danger. It is also known as bravery. Without courage, we cannot practice any other virtue with consistency. We can't be kind, true, merciful, generous, or honest". We are the real courageous voices of caregiving. We have more than a role. We have a calling. We should take pride in what we do. Sometimes we laugh so that we do not cry. Our lives are filled with many unknowns, and yet we continue to step forward and do what it takes to give the best care we can to our loved one. Each day our courage strengthens us. Like the lion in the <u>Wizard of Oz</u> our courage was always there, we just had to recognize it. We may be ordinary caregivers, but we have extraordinary courage.

I recognize my courage and take pride in it.

Prayer

Prayer is not something that can only be done in a church or a temple. We can pray with our eyes opened or closed or with our hands folded or open. It is said that you can pray in a closet, and God will hear you. Sometimes our prayers move us out of our comfort zone. We need to let go of our egos and trust that God's wisdom is greater than ours is. God's love is truth, and it will lead us to comfort and hope. No prayer is too big or too small. God will be the judge. He did not create us, then go off, and leave us to flounder on our own. He is always there. If we let go of the thought that we are the controller and surrender our will, many doors will be open. We will find peace and a sense of serenity that will carry us through the toughest times.

Today I will surrender myself to God and say,
"not my will, but yours"

Decision Time

There are times in our lives when we should not be making decisions. When we are under stress, angry or fatigued, we should never even entertain the thought of making a decision. At these times, we cannot think clearly or rationally. When we take time to make rational decisions, we allow ourselves the opportunity to gather the information and consider all alternatives that best suit our situation. It is difficult enough to make decisions for ourselves, but if we have to make them for a love one, we need to take extra precautions. We are more apt to make clearer judgments and better decisions if we are calm and take our time. The more information we have, the easier and more grounded our decisions will be. We cannot expect to have all the answers, and there may be a time when we need to call on others to guide us.

I will not make decisions in times of distress. I will take my time and weigh the odds.

Appreciation

Most of the time when we help people, they appreciate what we have done. They may even show their gratitude with a small gift or a note of thanks. If it were only that simple for our loved one to say thank you! Unfortunately, the help and care we give to our loved one cannot usually be expressed because they are unable to demonstrate their appreciation in words. Even though we know they cannot express their feelings, we sometimes ask ourselves "I wonder if they, or anyone else for that matter, really care about all the good I do?" We feel unloved and under appreciated. It's normal to feel that way at times as long as we don't wallow in our own self-pity. When we look deep inside our hearts, we know our loved one love us and that they would express it if they could.

I know I am loved and appreciated even when though my loved one cannot express it.

Caregiver Illness

When we are asked if we have gone to the doctors lately, we answer yes, but we are usually talking about our love one's doctor appointment. This is one of many ways we neglect ourselves. We know we should take better care of ourselves, but we just do not have the time. The fact is that if we are a spouse caregiver, we have a 35% chance of dying before our loved one. Our immune systems are being compromised, leaving us susceptible to many diseases. Our emotional state becomes shaky, leading us towards depression and other emotional illnesses. If we do not want to become a statistic, we need to care for ourselves properly and at times put ourselves first. Sacrificing our own health for our loved one makes no sense.

I will make a doctor's appointment for myself so that I can stay physically and emotionally healthy.

Pack Your Survival Kit

We know how important it is to care for our selves. We are grasping the concept, and now we need to take some preventative action. There will be times when we don't have time to prepare for what is happening. Having our legal and financial papers in order is a must! We need to list emergency contacts and formulate a plan that is ready to put into action. It is not enough for only ourselves to know what our plans are, or where our documents are located. We need to share this information with a family member or a trusted friend. These are the people that will most likely put our plan into action when we cannot. By expecting the unexpected, we can put things in order and have peace of mind.

I will review my emergency plans and documents, and share them with the people I have chosen to act upon them.

Resentment

We do not have to speak our resentment in order for it to affect others. Resentment is usually an accumulation of hurtful, negative thoughts that when held in, can fester and explode in a most inappropriate manner. These thoughts and feelings can cause great pain for our friends and family. When we have resentment, a major part of us shuts down, and we become bitter towards others and ourselves. We cannot always control how we feel about a person, but we can control how we respond to these feelings. Dealing with our resentments in a timely manner will help stop the festering of resentment and rid us of our toxic feelings. Rabbi Malachy McCourt says it so eloquently: "Resentment is like taking poison and waiting for the other person to die."

I will respond to my feeling in a timely manner so that they do not grow into resentment.

February 24

Fulfillment

We are so busy trying to survive that when we do have a break and have time to reflect, we often feel unfulfilled. Our personal lives have been put on hold, and taken a back seat to our caregiving. To feel fulfilled we must take a positive step and look at the question, "what would make me happy." It may be as simple as a new hairstyle or lunch out with a friend. Although these are baby steps toward feeling happy, they are a beginning. We need to step up to the plate and make the call and arrange for someone to care for our loved one, if only for a couple of hours. Then, we can go and do the happy thing that we so much want and deserve. It is amazing what this special time will do towards helping us feel content and fulfilled. Now that we are feeling better physically and mentally, we are ready to resume our role as caregiver.

I will take the baby step towards fulfillment so that
I can feel whole, and content.

Loyalty

Loyalty is love that endures throughout time. Married people have said it in their vows, "for better, for worse, for richer, for poorer". This disease can test our loyalty and our love. It takes an enormous commitment to offer ourselves as personal caregivers. This may not be the life we have chosen, but it is the life we have. What we do with it is up to us. In the beautiful story "The Notebook" by Nicolas Sparks we get to see what enduring, faithful love is. The husband's love does not falter even as he struggle with the reality of his wife's Alzheimer's. Like the character in "The Notebook", our love is non-ending and we remain devoted and dedicated to our loved one. We give our selfless love in hopes that we can make their days better. We can stand tall knowing that we have been loyal to the end.

I will remain steadfast and give my loved one enduring love.

Rosie the Riveter

During WW11, there were posters of Rosie the Riveter, flexing her arm muscle, and the poster read, "We can do it". It grabbed the attention of women all over America, and they stepped up to take the place of the men in factories that had gone to war. Like the women of the 40s, we have stepped up to take care of our loved one. With purposeful action, we meet the challenges of caring for someone with Alzheimer's. We have been called on to make a difference, and their well-being depends on us. The life of our loved one is in our hands, and we will give them all we have. Our caregiving is a testament of our spirit, and we give of it freely and with love.

I will care for my loved one with an open heart and fulfill their needs whenever possible.

Free Time

Yearning free time is almost an adult pastime, yet we believe free time is unattainable. Is it the lack of time that is the problem, or is it the lack of will to create the time? Time management sounds so staunch, but if we look at it as making a plan and following through with it, our goal becomes more palatable and attainable. Free time does not have to be measured in increments of hours. Some of our greatest pleasures can be found in moments. Smelling freshly brewed coffee, seeing the first robin of spring, watching the trees burst with color in autumn, can delight our senses. There really is time for us to use for our pleasure. We just need to find it. Looking for free time only in large blocks, can rob us of these sweet cherished moments.

I will manage my time so that I can enjoy the many
pleasures that surround me.

Never Say Never

The word "never" carries a lot of negative power. It is a word we use to communicate to others and ourselves exactly how we feel. I will never treat my loved one like that. I will never put them in a nursing home. These are strong statements that in the future could come back to haunt us. Never has a binding effect that makes it hard for us to make a decision when presented with personal decisions dealing with our loved one. The old saying "never say never" is so true. Never is a very long time, and it does not take into consideration that time and circumstances change. Our health status or financial conditions can change in an instant causing us to change our best-laid plans. We can still feel strongly about something and hope that it never happens. This is not so much a Pollyanna approach as it is common sense.

I will refrain from using "Never" when making decisions.

Up Side of Days

"The rising and falling waves may drown us, or wash us to shore, depending on how we ride them." This is a wise and prophetic saying. How we do each day depends on how we use it. If we rise and think this day has no redeeming features and with nothing good to look forward to, then it will become true. Of course, it is not enough to think it is going to be a good day; we need to act on it. Thinking about how we can do things smarter thus making them easier, will help us get through some of the toughest times. By keeping our days on an even keel, we will be better prepared to ride the waves. We can accomplish more when we feel better emotionally and have more quality time to enjoy. Our days truly are what we make them.

I will greet each day with the positive affirmation;
Today is going to be a great day.

March

∾

"I've learned that people will forget what you said, people will forget what you did, but people will never forget how you made them feel."

Maya Angelou

The Battle

Erin Brocovitch took on the battle for the people of Hinkley who could not do it for themselves. We need to take on the battle for our loved one, "who would if they could." We need to advocate for them in many ways. They deserve to be treated with respect and dignity. When they go to the hospital, the same loving care received by a child should be theirs also. People need to understand that our loved one is a viable person that, before their illness, was a doctor, lawyer, the mother, or fathers. They took their place in society and made it a better place to live. If we need to shout it from the rooftops, "treat them kindly, they are not their disease". There is no need for them to have second best.

I will stand up for my loved one and assure that they never have to settle for second best.

Rudeness

Rudeness is never acceptable, but it is sometimes understandable. There are days when we feel like nothing can go right. The least little thing can set us off. Everyone has these types of days, but it is not an excuse to lash out and be rude to others. We may try to make an excuse for our actions by believing that we were just trying to be honest or that the person deserved what they got. When we are rude to people, we denigrate them and ourselves. Rudeness is also used as a defense mechanism, a type of self-defense if you will, that stops others from getting too close. We rationalize that we need to get them before they get us. We usually do not do this out of disrespect for others. We do not mean to be rude, but sometimes our mouth speaks before our brain engages.

I will think before I speak so that I will show
respect for others and myself.

Exercise

We know how important exercise is for our health and well-being. It is equally important for our loved one. Exercise can have many benefits. Not only can it help them sleep better, it can also help during periods of agitation. There is no need to work out to Richard Simons' "Sweaten to the Oldies". Simple walking together is enough. Walking can also be invigorating as well giving us some special time together. This simple form of exercise can be tailored to all levels of functions. On bad weather days, a stroll through the mall will be a nice change of pace. If walking is not an option, simple chair exercises work very well. When we exercise with them, it is more fun for them and good for us. Moving at their pace and not rushing can make these times special and fulfilling.

I will set up an exercise program that will work
for my loved one as well as me.

March 4

Promises

Who among us caregivers hasn't made the well-meaning promise, 'I will never put you in a nursing home", or "I will always take care of you"/ As the primary or secondary caregiver, we meant what we said at the time. We felt there was nothing that could stop us from caring for our loved one until the end. As the disease progresses, we may be finding that their needs are more than we can handle, yet we still hear the echo of the promise and try to abide by it. We try whatever we can to keep them at home until a crisis with them or our own health is in such a decline that the promise must be broken. This is another situation where emotions take over and blur our judgment. As difficult as it may be, we must begin to lay the groundwork so that we are prepared if that day comes.

I will keep an open mind, and if I must break my promise,
I will know that I have done the best I could.

Limiting Attitudes

"Well, that's just the way I am" is almost never a valid justification for how we live our lives. By arguing our limitations, we create our own hurdles. We also believe that we must act accordingly no matter what others think of us. Believing such self-serving statements will put limitations on us leaving no room for growth. Psychologists say that we tend to do what we tell ourselves to do. Some things are more difficult for us, but that does not mean we cannot change. We have the capacity to learn and change. Having a "can-do-it" attitude is an exceptional quality that helps us overcome whatever difficulties we may have. We cannot let limiting attitudes take over our life. We can master challenges, overcome obstacles, and be in control of our life if we are willing to try.

I will build on my can-do attitude so that I can face any challenges that come before me.

March 6

Fairness of Life

Is life fair? That is the proverbial question. It is probably safe to say life is not always fair. Life did not seem fair when we got the diagnosis of Alzheimer's, but it did seem fair when we won the trip to Hawaii. Maybe life is not meant to be fair. If it were, bad things would not happen to good people. On the other hand, maybe life is fair. The challenges that are set before us give us the opportunity to make things better. Probably the best answer is life does not always seem fair. Just because we do not always get what we want doesn't make life unfair. In times like these, we need to find value in the moment. We cannot take the disease away, but we can make our loved one's life better. Life is what we make it. If we see it as unfair, that is a sign of giving up. Life is a gift... it depends on how we use it.

I will cherish the gift of life and live it to my potential, for life is what I make it.

Organization

There are times when we wish that we were as organized as our friend, or maybe we have seen a TV show where someone comes into the home and organizes it for them, and we wish that person would show up at our door. Now the job of organizing may seem overwhelming, but we can do it using small increments of time. We can begin by making a list of the spaces that bother us the most. Each time we organize them, we can check them off the list. This will simplify our life and give us a great feeling of accomplishment. Just doing a drawer a day can make us feel more in control. This definitely is an area of our life, over which we have control. While organizing, it is a good idea to put away things that could present a safety issue. By keeping our surroundings minimalist, we will feel less stress and will not have to worry about where we put things.

I will set mini goals for organizing and follow the plan.

$P_{riorities}$

We can look back in our earlier years when we prided ourselves for having the cleanest house in the neighborhood. Now we just cannot seem to get caught up. In the earlier years, we may have been a little more structured and life seemed a little easier. Now that we are caregivers, our life does not really have any structure, and we do not know what will happen from minute to minute. We try to duo-task just to stay afloat. It is difficult to plan for something, because we never know how our loved one will be that day. Unrealistic priorities can cause stress and put us over the top. We should never be so proud that we refuse to ask for help. Just having someone pick our clothes up from the cleaners can give us more time to do the things we need to do.

I will reassess my priorities and learn to ask for help.

Play

Play is not just for children. Wouldn't it be fun to set a play date just for ourselves? We could have a day where we did not have to care for anyone but ourselves. For one day, we could do away with all the things that are constantly competing for our time and energy. We could call a friend, go to a movie, and eat all the junk food we want. Maybe, we could go to the beach or take a ride to an old favorite haunt. It does not have to make sense; it just has to be fun. What we do does not matter as much as how we do it. We need to play with a carefree attitude. The only thing that matters is us. We let go of our structured day and do only what we want to do. We play, laugh, and feel joy in just being ourselves. So let's not just think about it, "let's do it."

I will set a play date for myself and recapture the joy I knew as a child.

Cure

At this time there are no medications that can cure Alzheimer's. Even though there is no cure, some drugs can help slow the progression. The jury is out on agreement about how helpful these drugs are. If we are going to error, then let us do so on the positive side. The thought of having even a little more quality in their lives is worth reaching for. Attention should also be paid to exercise and diet, and we should take into consideration other illness they may also have. Because there is no cure, we need to hedge our bet by doing all we can to insure the quality of life they deserve. Along with their health needs, doing meaningful activities and gentle exercise, we may be able to slow their decline. Who knows what the future may hold? A break through could happen at any time, and we need to be ready.

*I will look at all options that will help my loved
one have a better quality of life.*

Safety

Creating a safe environment for our loved one is very important. Their lives are filled with obstacles. They may not be able to see the throw rugs that we have decorated with through out the house. Stoves and hot water become dangerous because they no longer know how to use or regulate them. There are many things we can do to make our homes safer. We can start by taking an inventory of our home and removing things that could be hazardous to them. We should look beyond the obvious, and child proof our home as if we had a toddler running around. They can see things like buttons lying on a table as food, and thus they will put them into their mouth. Things that we would normally keep under the sink need to be removed. By taking these safety measures early, we can prevent falls and other life threatening injuries.

Today I will take an inventory of my house and do what is necessary to keep my loved one safe.

Name

We show our respect to others in many ways. The Latin root of respect means, "To look again" and this is what needs to happen with our loved one. People need to look again, past their disease and into who and what they are. A person's sense of who they are is closely connected to the name they are commonly called by. Their sense of identity is already being compromised, without people referring to them as honey, sweetie, or darling. Because of their decline, they feel vulnerable and name recognition is very important. Our names were given to us out of love at our birth, and we all have the right and the need to be addressed by our name. What is in a name? It could be self worth or just name recognition. Whatever it is, this is one of the ways that others show them and us the respect we all deserve.

I will help others know the preferred name of my loved one, so that they can address them with respect.

Silence

Sometimes silence can be so loud. We do not think of silence as necessarily a good thing. Our fast moving world is so noise filled, that we become uneasy in the face of silence. By nature, we are not solitary creatures and silence makes us uneasy. We even think that something is wrong because we are desensitized to the noise around us. It is a pity that we fear silence. Learning to be comfortable with silence is learning to be comfortable with ourselves. Being able to cultivate our inner silence is one of the greatest tools we can give to ourselves. Silence truly can be golden if we use it for quiet moment of reflection. It can take us places where we can listen to our heart and see the many opportunities and blessings we really have.

*I will greet silence with anticipation and reflect
on the good in my life.*

Progression

In the beginning they may have known their memory was failing and even attempted to hide it. As they progressed, they needed simple assistance but began to dismiss the idea that they were having memory problems. They then moved into a stage where they needed almost total care. This is usually when, if there is any merciful point in the progression of this disease, it is that they cannot remember what they have forgotten. They have no awareness of the problems and begin to disconnect from most all their sensory information. The latter stages are probably sadder for us than they are for them. They appear to have less stress and have a more child like demeanor about them. Their memory and reasoning are failing, but their need for our unconditional love is needed now more than ever.

Today I will show my unconditional love in all that I do for my loved one.

Ask for Help

Asking for help is not a weakness, but we as caregivers are infamous for trying to do everything for ourselves. People really want to help but often do not know what to do. It could be as simple as asking someone to make an extra serving of their delicious spaghetti sauce so that we can put it in our freezer for a day when we are just too tired to cook. It is ok to ask someone to spend a couple of hours with our loved one, so that we can get a much-needed break. We should not rob people of the opportunity to help. People have good hearts and want to help us. They just need a little guidance to know what to do. Help can come in many forms. It could be something as simple as a friend asking, "Could I pick something up for you" I am going to the store. Someone stopping by and giving us a sympathetic ear can be a great help. Sometimes it is the simplest things that help us the most.

I will learn how to ask for help and ask for what I need.

March 16

Procrastination

We were going to organize our papers but just did not get around to it. We have the missing button to our shirt, but we do not seem to remember to sew it on until we want to wear it, and then there really is not time to do it. Procrastination costs us a lot of grief. We spend a great deal of time thinking about what needs to be done, instead of doing it. Most often, the problem with procrastinating is that we just cannot seem to get started. The task often seems too big to start or too small to worry about it. When we do not do things that need to be done in a timely manner, we waste a lot of time worrying about them and put even more stress upon ourselves. There is great satisfaction in doing things now. By not putting things off, we can accomplish more in less time and have a feeling of accomplishment.

I will not put off until tomorrow what I can do today.

Reminiscence

Webster's dictionary defines reminiscing as the act of recalling past events or experiences. At one time it was thought that it was only a musing of the frail elderly. It is so much more that that. It can be a life affirming activity that can help us review happy times and events. It also has a benefit to our health by slowing us down and reducing our stress. Of course, we will remember some not so good things, but hopefully we have learned from our past mistakes. Recalling our accomplishments makes us feel good and is good for our self-image. Sharing pictures or stories of the past is also a positive thing to do with our loved one. It may also help us have a more positive interaction with them. Reminiscing can also provide us with comfort and consolation when we are facing a loss. With any luck, we will remember more good things than bad.

I will use reminiscing to awaken the memories that I have stored in my soul.

Excuses

Too often we get comfortable with where we are, and use our circumstances as a caregiver as a crutch. "I can't, I don't have time, and it's not fun anymore." We also use excuses for not joining a support group: "I'm not a group type of person, I can't leave my loved one, I can't talk to strangers." We begin to take steps towards total isolation and our social life begins to fade. It is true, it does take longer to get our loved one ready to go out, but that is not an excuse not to go. "He doesn't eat much these days," is not a reason to stop making nutritious meals. We get stuck in the label of the disease and only see what we cannot do instead of what we can do. This role as a caregiver is only one part of who we are as a complete person. We need to nurture all aspects of ourselves: physical, spiritual, mental, and emotional. This includes knowing our limitations, taking time for ourselves, asking for and accepting support. We need to keep doing the things we enjoy, so we do not become resentful of the demands that caregiving places on us.

I will not define myself by this disease but will nurture my body and my soul.

Death

The day we are born, we begin to die. As harsh, as it sounds it is true. Most families have an unwritten rule; we do not talk about death. We all wish that death would come to our loved one in the quiet of the night as we sleep. The truth is this is not usually the way it happens. Although we do not have a choice as to when we die, we do have some choices as to how we want to be cared for when we are dying. As difficult as it is, end of life choices should be a topic that all families talk about. If our loved one is too far along in their disease process, it may be too late to discuss it with them, but it is not too late for us to make our wishes known. If we prepare for our last days as carefully as we prepare for the present, we can take our leave with dignity.

I will speak with my family about how I wish to be cared for when my time comes.

Beauty

There is a song that is sung in the Unity Church that proclaims, "If you think that God doesn't hear you, then listen with your eyes." We need to take a moment and step outside, get some fresh air and look at nature all around us. When we see the clouds floating by, the flowers, the majestic trees, and the carefree birds, we surely must know that these are not the creation of man, but those of a higher power, who really listens to us. There is no denying that a mortal man is not capable of such creations. Even in the eighteen hundreds John Muir, a naturalist, knew of the beauty of nature and its healing powers. Muir observes, "Nature's peace will flow into you as sunshine flows into trees. The winds will blow their own freshness into you... while cares will drop off like autumn." When we ask for something and do not get the answer we want right away, it is easy to think that God has not heard us. It is at these times we need to reflect on the beauty around us and remember that God is in charge of all. His answers will come in His time.

*I will open my eyes and ears to God's creations
and enjoy their beauty.*

Personal Health

Making our personal health a priority has to be at the top of our "to do list". It is not enough to just be on the list, we must act on it. There is never an excuse as to why we cannot or do not do it. The adverse consequences of not caring for ourselves are well documented. Health is more than health of the body. It also means health of mind and soul. If we wait to take care of ourselves until we are brought to our knees, there will be a high price to pay. It is not selfish to focus on our needs its part of our job. This thing we call caregiving is a true balancing act, wherein we have many balls in the air at the same time. If we drop all the balls who will be there to pick them up? We cannot allow ourselves to be the second victim. If we neglect our health, we many end up so ill that we have to stop caring for our loved one. Who will care for them then? Just worrying about our health is not enough. Every day we need to take time out to develop and nurture ourselves.

I will make my personal health a priority
and take action to assure it.

Rituals

Simple every day acts can be comfortable rituals. A warm cup of coffee before we begin our busy day is a simple but soothing ritual. Rituals can be very important because they help us to become grounded. Rituals can also be helpful to our loved one. Taking a short walk hand-in-hand, having a cup of warm cocoa when the first days of winter arrives, can give a feeling of love and comfort to us both. We may have forgotten some of the rituals we used to enjoy together, or we may choose not to remember them. Our busy schedules seem to take over our actions, but we have the ability to reinstate some of our most loved rituals. We can do this by slowing down our pace and thinking about what gives meaning to us now. Rediscovering our comforting rituals can help us bring clarity into our lives, and we will be able to enjoy the simple things.

I will re-establish the rituals that gave
us comfort and joy in the past.

Starting Our Day

Our thoughts are initiators of our actions. So where will our thoughts take us today? Will I let myself be overwhelmed by all that I have to do, or will I work smarter and use my positive plan of action? In experiencing a fresh new day we can let go of our negative thoughts and open ourselves to the positive side of caring. By taking the time each morning to set our priorities and ask for guidance, we can move on in our day in a positive manner. Our days can also be more enjoyable and fulfilling when we approach them with optimism. Having something to look forward to, no matter how small it may be, lifts our spirits, gives us confidence and makes getting out of bed each morning worthwhile.

Today is full of possibilities. I will keep a positive attitude and look forward to this God-given day.

March 24

What Do You Do

There is a question that may be rude, but it is asked often; so what do you do? Our Answer could be "Oh I am just a caregiver". We have just insulted ourselves when we down played our role as caregiver. There is no such thing as just a caregiver. Let us look at the many hats that caregivers wear, and examine the breath of the care we give. We are cooks, housekeepers, personal shopper, nurse, laundryman, psychologist, transportation specialist, hygienist, maintenance manager, companion and these are just a few of our responsibilities. So if we are feeling tired, we have good reason to be. We do the jobs that most people would not even consider doing and we do it all, in the name of love. The next time someone rudely asks us "so what do you do?" let us reply, "I am a courageous caregiver extraordinaire."

I am proud of my role as caregiver and I will let others know the magnitude of my job.

Caregivers Just the Same

Just because we do not live in the same house as our loved one, perhaps they are in a nursing home, does not make us any less a caregiver. In fact, advocating for our loved one or trying to do things from a distance presents its own challenges. Caregiver worries seem to magnify when we cannot be with them every moment. We are not with them at these times not because we do not want to be but because our life at this time does not allow it. We are busy negotiating their care and advocating for their rights. We locate and coordinate their care. Decisions have to be made and finances have to be monitored. We are the negotiators and delegates who ensure the welfare of our loved one. Beyond a doubt, we are caregivers personified and we do make a difference in their life.

I will take pride in my caregiver duties, and make the decisions I need to make with confidence.

March 26

Healthy Brains

We know that we need to take care of ourselves physically, but it is also very important to keep our brains active and healthy. We think, "I don't have time for silly games or crossword puzzles." Even though we have heard this cry before we need to recognize that it really is, "a use it or lose it" situation. Science tells us that by keeping the brain active we may be able to increase its vitality and possibly generate new brain cells. Researchers have also found that what is good for the heart is good for the brain. Foods high in anti-oxidants combined with exercise and mental stimulation helps maintain a healthy brain. There is no proof that all this will stop us from getting Alzheimer's, but it has been proven that living a brain healthy life style will help keep us mentally alert and active.

I will seek out stimulating activities so that
I can keep my brain healthy.

Hospice

The very mention of the word hospice puts fear in most caregivers. We think of the H word as being a death sentence. "If we have hospice, they will let them die." By accepting the reality of what is happening in the later stages of the disease, we can better see death as a natural part of life. Hospice is a concept that focuses on the quality and dignity of life by providing comfort to our loved one, as well as to their family. More than the fear of death, we fear the possibility of pain in death. In the end stages, our loved one may suffer multiple problems such as heart disease or pneumonia. It is probable that we will know when hospice is needed before our doctor does. We need to act as their advocate and ask our doctor to request this end of life care. This has been a long journey, and we can fulfill our loved one's wishes by treasuring life and respecting death.

I treasure and respect life, and when the end grows near I will look to hospice for comfort care.

Circular thinking

Sometimes we feel as though we are stuck in a rut. We re-hash the same things over and over. Our minds get stuck in a vicious thought cycle. Most often we do not emerge with any resolution. It goes something like this: "I don't have time to look for in home help. I couldn't afford it if I did find it. They probably wouldn't be able to help that much anyway." Circulr thinking is an ineffective way of problem solving. We literally go in circles. We become self defeating, afraid to make decisions or try new things. When a dog chases his tail, has he won when he catches, it or was it just something to do at the moment? Circular thinking makes us re-hash things over and over again without a viable solution.

I will stop re-hashing my old thoughts, so that I don't get stuck in circular thinking.

Happiness

We want to be happy, but we seem to look for it in all the wrong places. We believe that if we just have more money or a better job we will be happy. We believe that we need to earn happiness or look towards others for our happiness. We often fixate on what is bad and get stuck in a negative time frame. When we look outside ourselves for happiness, we become our own worst enemy. The truth is that happiness comes from within. Yes, we will sometimes be sad or hurt, but these times are a normal part of life, once we accept them we can gracefully move on towards our true happiness. There is really no definition for happiness because it is different for everybody; it is a state of mind. Happiness is a choice. It is up to us to cultivate it. Dale Carnegie tells us: "Remember, happiness doesn't depend upon who you are or what you have: it depends solely on what you think."

I will search within myself for happiness
and not depend on others.

Emotions

In the period of one day, we deal with many emotions. Some may be soft and compassionate and others harsh and angry. Our emotions are embedded in our minds, but we still have control over them. Our emotions drive our behavior, in other words we are the rulers of our destiny. Sometimes our feelings get the best of us, leading us to act irrationally and illogically. Our emotions are also an important means by which we evaluate situations and make decisions about what is appropriate in a given situation. Unchecked emotions tend to lead us to impulsive behavior. How we chose to act upon the emotion is strictly up to us, but if we choose to cultivate emotional balance, we will be better equipped to handle our daily demands.

I will be conscious of my emotions and
approach decisions rationally.

Stigma

Alzheimer's is hard to say and more difficult to spell, and people just do not want to talk about it. Like the proverbial ostrich, if we do not see it, it is not there, and it probably will not happen to us any way. It's a terrible disease that only happens to other people. It has a stigma attached to it that is so strong that it often delays diagnosis for up to six years. As caregivers, we know that some people treat us differently once our loved one has the diagnosis. Most stigmas are often caused by lack of knowledge. There is not enough public awareness, and people just do not want to hear about it. "There but for the grace of God there go I." If we are to erase this stigma, we must be willing to share our knowledge and advocates for all that are stricken with it. As we know, knowledge is power.

*I will use my knowledge of this disease
to help erase its stigma.*

April

~

*See how nature - trees, flowers, grass — grows
in silence; see the stars, the moon and the sun,
how they move in silence...we need silence to be
able to touch souls.*

MOTHER TERESA

.

Personal Gratitude

In our hectic and busy lives as caregiver, we sometimes lose sight of the things that are positive in our lives. When we worry or become upset over things, we make them appear bigger than they really are. Negativity attracts negativity. By focusing on what is good in our lives, we leave little room for things that are not. Gratitude is a great remedy for a whole lot of problems. By expressing gratitude, we are giving a gift to others and ourselves. By slowing down and reflecting on the things, we are grateful for, we will begin to lead a more positive life. Gratitude is the equalizer in life that says, "life owes me nothing, and the good in my life is a gift." Gratitude helps us truly enjoy and appreciate life. Did our loved one smile at us today? Now that is something to be grateful about.

*I will focus on all the good in my life and
give thanks for what I have.*

Taking Time

Taking time to think about it, or, as Oprah says "taking time to pray on it", refers to the time we need to take before making big decisions. Very little in life demands that we act upon something immediately. Decisions that are made in haste often come back to haunt us. Yes, we are people pleasers and have a hard time saying no. We want to do what others ask of us, even when we know we should not. Our society tries to get us to make snap decisions: "This offer is only good for one day, week, or hour." What good or service is so great that it has a time limit on it? Decisions like these are made through impulsive thinking. Taking time to think it out, or "pray on it" will help us make the right decision for our loved one and us.

I will not make snap decisions. I will take the time needed to make informed decisions.

Smart Prayer

Sometimes we pray and pray about something, and we just do not get an answer. Maybe we need to be more trusting in our prayers. It is like asking question after question and not giving the person time to answer. God does hear us the first time around, and we need to have faith that he will answer. Our timetable is not the same as God's, because we are usually driven to prayer by fear, want, or anxiety. Everything has a gestation period; we just need to give it time to come forward. We pray for "God's will be done", not ours. It is all right to pray about something more than once, but we must also realize that time gives faith time to grow. To put things in perspective, it took 120 years for the flood to come so Noah could use his ark. Not only was that patience, but it was also faith.

I have faith that my prayers will be answered in God's time not mine.

Love and Respect

It is said that we make a living by what we get, but we make a life by what we give. Being caregivers, we are good at this caregiving thing. There is however one question we need to ask ourselves. Are we giving out of the spirit of love or out of a sense of duty? Do we merely exist in this caregiver roll because someone has to do it? The attitude we attach to our caregiving can affect the way we deliver care. Doing something only because we feel we are forced to can render us uncaring and callous. Doing something out of love and respect can help us and our loved one feel fulfilled and content. This is the best care of all. It reflects the goodness and devotion we have for our loved one. It also puts people on notice that this is how you expect them to treat us.

I will care for my loved one out of devotion
and love and be the best I can be.

Helping Others

We have a unique opportunity to help others. We have "walked the walk" and can "talk the talk". There is not much another caregiver can tell us that would be a shock. Other caregivers will look to us for wisdom, knowledge and support. By remembering what it felt like on our early journey, we can help steady them and let them know that they can do this. Fledging caregivers will make mistakes just as we did, but with our support, they will learn from them as we did. We are caregivers and our compassion for others is strong. We have empathy and understand their struggle. The greatest gift we can give to them is to listen in their time of need.

*I will be there for other caregivers and share
my knowledge and support with them.*

April 6

Vacations

Right now, a vacation is something we did years ago and probably with our loved one. We would not think of taking one without them. We know we need time to ourselves, but a vacation is out of the question. We would feel guilty. No one can care for them as we can. What if something happened while we were gone? Our concerns stem from the illusion that if we are there with them, nothing bad can happen. We feel the need to be in complete control. If we plan well, there is no reason we cannot take a few days for ourselves. We need to get away and refocus. We need freedom from our daily environment, and we need to interact with other people. By getting away and enjoying ourselves, we will improve our own mental health and come back refreshed so that we can continue to be the amazing caregivers we are.

In an effort to refocus and refresh, I will plan some personal leisure time for myself.

One More Day

Mitch Albom in his book "For One More Day" asks the question "What if we had one more day with our loved one?" If we had only one more day with our loved one, it would not matter that their clothes do not match or that they have food stains on their shirt. It would not make any difference that they cannot remember something that just happened. The soiled bedding or the mess at the table would not even faze us. What would matter is that in many ways they are still with us. Their smile, the sound of their voice, the way they look at us when they feel safe and content in our presence, are what really matters. Our whole outlook on life and the way we live it would come down to the simple things, if we only had one more day.

I will give thanks for the days I still have with my loved one, for each day is a treasured gift.

Family Dynamics

Our family dynamics dictate the role we play in our family, how we communicate, and what our boundaries are within the family. This is neither good nor bad, but it does affect how we work with others throughout our life. If we were able to be open and flexible in our early family life, we will be better able to cope with problems that occur in our later life. How we express ourselves has much to do with what we learned from our families as we were growing up. How we resolve conflict or solve problems is directly related to this learned behavior. In order to have our families assist us in our caregiving, we will need to evaluate what our family dynamics are and how to best approach the caregiving issue with them so that we are heard and acknowledged.

I will evaluate my family dynamics before I approach my family for help.

Centering Ourselves

We often hear the phrase "centering yourself" in conjunction with yoga or meditation. Simply put, centering is taking the time to be in the moment. When we stop, think, and take a deep breath, we are centering ourselves. In fact we probably center ourselves frequently. When we are faced with a tough decision, we calm ourselves and focus on making the best decision possible. When we need to slow the pace of our day, we stop and regroup our thoughts. When we are upset with our loved one and want to argue, or fear we are going to say something we should not, centering ourselves is a good solution. If we practice centering ourselves, we will be better prepared to take positive actions in a negative situation. This is a powerful way to process our every day problems.

I will find a way to center myself so that I can be up for any challenge I face.

Integrity

To live with integrity means to live in accordance with our beliefs and standards. It is doing the right thing and not yielding to the temptation of taking the easy way out. It sometimes can be hard to hold on to our integrity. There may have been times when we have yielded to the easy way thus compromising our integrity, only to find it really was not worth it. We know in our hearts what is right, and yet we sometimes side step it. Most of the time the small voice of our conscious will lead us in the right direction. We can rationalize all we want but in the end, integrity should win out. The author and philanthropist W. Clement Stone eloquently speaks of life with integrity: "Have the courage to say no. have the courage to face the truth. Do the right thing because it is right. These are the magic keys to living your life with integrity."

I will live my life with integrity and have
the courage to face the truth.

Criticism

Most people do not take criticism very well. We tend to take criticism as a direct attack against us. Sometimes it may not be just the criticism that makes us angry; it also can be the state of mind we are in when it is happens. If we are feeling bad about ourselves in the moment of criticism, it will only reinforce the negative feelings. Sometimes it is good to consider the source. There are people who are negative most of the time, and their criticism usually does not hold much credibility. No one can make us feel bad about our selves unless we let them. There are times when criticism is given to us in a constructive way, and we need to evaluate it. It will serve no purpose to become defensive or confrontational. There are battles that are just not worth fighting.

I will evaluate criticism and refrain from being defensive or confrontational.

April 12

Listening

In communicating with our loved one, listening is the most important element because it takes more time for them to formulate their thoughts and words. This is when we need to stop and really listen. We can't listen when we are talking. We need to be sensitive to their frustrations of not being able to convey their thoughts. We should listen and communicate patiently, and try to reduce the frustration they may feel from not being able to communicate effectively. If patience were ever a virtue, it is now when we are trying to meet their needs. Our goal is to understand not just their words, but also the meaning they are trying to get across. If they are making negative statements, we should not respond, and we should not take them personally. By truly listening, we can improve communication and can even calm negative behavior.

I will truly listen to my loved one so that I can communicate with them in the most efficient manner.

Blaming Others

It is human nature to blame someone at one time or another. Unfortunately, when we do this, we are not accepting our own personal responsibility. We are saying, "You are at fault, and I am not." It is an escape mechanism that will eventually backfire on us. There may even be times when it is someone else's fault, but if we dwell on it, we again become the victim. This doesn't mean we have to go through life letting other people walk all over us. When we feel confident in ourselves, there is no need to place blame. We are bigger than that, and we have better things to do with our life. We have the power within ourselves to make things happen. We become personally accountable for all that we do. Robert Anthony says, "When we blame others, we give up our power to change."

I will stop blaming others and take back my power.

Ownership of Feelings

Our feelings are 100% ours. No one can make us feel a certain way. We may say, "They made me feel this way", but this is not really so. It is our response to something that makes us feel a certain way, not the person or thing that causes the response. Our feelings are a response to our emotions, and only we can control them. When we take ownership of our feeling, we are giving ourselves control over them. Our feelings are like energetic forces that require us to take action. Through ownership, we gain control. When we have control of our feelings, we have the choice to change them. Ownership is the positive way of controlling how we feel and what we do with these feelings.

I will take ownership of my feelings so that I can have control over my emotions.

Permission

Giving ourselves permission to feel what we feel is sometimes very difficult. We are filled with so many mixed emotions that we often dismiss them thinking we should not feel that way. Some negative thoughts we think when we are angry or frustrated are perfectly normal and need to be recognized. It is ok to feel bad or frustrated we are only human. Sometimes we just need to let it out. If we do not acknowledge these feelings, we cannot move on. Our emotions will be up and down throughout our caregiver journey. If we continue to hold things in, we will eventually burn out. We must give ourselves permission to examine our feelings if we are going to deal with them.

I acknowledge that my feelings are valid, and I give myself permission to deal with them.

Optimism

Optimism is viewing life in a positive manner. Optimists generally believe that people and happenings are inherently good, and that all things happen for a reason. When we are optimistic, we believe that we can do something positive to make our situation better. We can do this because we are willing to take the action necessary to make it happen. Optimism is a self-fulfilling prophecy. We think and act in a positive manner, thus good things happen. When we harness the power of optimism, we also help reduce our stress. Winston Churchill knew about optimism and wrote, "A pessimist sees difficulty in every opportunity; an optimist sees opportunity in every difficulty". Our optimism lets us rise above the problem and see the good in others and our life.

I will rise above my problem and approach
the solution with optimism.

Status Quo

It is hard to watch our loved one age before their time. We watch as they grow helpless, confused, physically and mentally frail. We try to adjust to the changes and act like everything is status quo. Were afraid that if we give into their fragility, we will be betraying them and deny them their due respect. Some days are more difficult than others are. We are aware that their frailty makes them more likely to suffer from complications from even the simplest of ailments. A cold could send them into pneumonia. When things are not right, our days seem to go on forever, but the disease still progresses swiftly. We cannot stop the progression, but we can make a difference. In caring for them with love, we show our respect. We are their "knight in shining armor". Our love is in our actions.

I will stay alert to my loved one's frailty and
be there in their time of need.

April 18

Comforts of Home

Dorothy in the <u>Wizard of Oz</u> was not alone in her feelings of "there's no place like home". Just about everyone knows this feeling. Home represents comfort for us, a place where we take refuge and surround ourselves with family and familiar things. We slip into comfortable routines and are quieted with a feeling of wholeness. Our loved one cannot always explain what makes them feel comfortable and secure, but our knowledge of their past will help us know their comfort zone. Being surrounded with familiar things and using comfortable routines can help them feel secure and content. For the most part their needs are pretty basic. Like us, they want to feel the comfort and warmth our homes represent.

I will surround my loved one with the comforts of home,
even if we are not there.

Taking Things for Granted

If we have learned anything from this disease, it is not to take anything for granted. Our days can change hourly. What worked yesterday may not work today. As much as we would like to have a good workable routine, that is not always in the cards either. Although this sounds bad, it is not all that terrible. Life would be pretty boring if all things remained the same. This disease has taught us to appreciate the small things. We have learned how to cherish things that others do not even see. Life is so precious to us now. Each day that we have to spend with our loved one is a gift. We are learning to bend and sway with change. "You never know what you have until it's gone", hopefully this saying will not be true in our life. The eloquence of G.K. Chesterton's quote should guide us, "When it comes to life the critical thing is whether you take things for granted or take them with gratitude."

I will stop taking things for granted and start taking them with gratitude.

Escape

There are many ways to escape the realities of our life, and some of them are not good. We all need some Calgon moments, but how we obtain them is the key. A drink here, a pill there, could lead to another and another and that is where the line is drawn. Yes, we feel better for the moment, but if we continue to use these avenues of escape, we are setting ourselves up for disaster. The guilt we feel from an addiction far out weighs the momentary relief. We need to monitor our behavior as well as that of our loved one. If we see ourselves moving towards an unhealthy life style, we need to seek professional help. Our behavior is controllable; our loved one's is not. We need to embrace life not escape it.

I will monitor my modes of escape and work towards a healthier lifestyle.

Treadmill of Life

What a hurried society we live in! We rush here and there, sometimes only to sit and wait. We cannot continue to keep going full speed ahead. Slowing our lives down to a manageable pace can be difficult, but it is necessary. Our daily activities with our loved one cannot go at a break neck speed. Their world needs to be calm and slow. Their brains cannot process things that come at them too fast. Limiting our activities to doing one thing at a time will help slow down the pace. Slowing ourselves down can be difficult, but since we set the pace for our loved one, it is necessary that we do so. We can no longer live our lives on a treadmill because no matter how fast we go we will never get there. "Never before have we had so little time in which to do so much." Franklin D. Roosevelt recognize this problem way back in the late nineteen forties.

I will slow my daily life down to a manageable pace and get off the treadmill of life.

April 22

Competition

Competition may be good for business or sports, but it has no place in our relations with our family. When we are in competition with someone, our goal is to win at any expense. We try to prove that we are right and they are wrong, or that we can do something better than they can. The problem with this line of action is we both lose. We each become more entrenched in being right or winning resulting in hurt feelings or broken relationships. Families are torn apart, and often we are unable to reconcile. If this has happened in our family, we need to stand up and try to fix it. If we look back at what the reasons are for this distancing, it is a good bet we cannot remember what they were. Relationships are not a game; family is too precious to let words and hurt egos break it apart. We should never build the wall so high that we cannot get over it.

I will work on my relationship with my family and recognize the good that we have together.

Paranoia

Along with the memory loss, we may also experience a sense of paranoia in our loved one. They may think we are stealing from them, or that someone is after them. Their confused world can turn into a nightmare. As crazy as this sound, it is very real in their world. In a state of paranoia, they can become frustrated and scared. What is a caregiver to do? First, we can acknowledge their feelings. We also know never to argue with them. If they think there is a man under their bed, then there is. Sometimes a simple reassuring touch or simple redirecting will be enough. However, we always need to validate what they say, and then we can pretend to get rid of the scoundrel. There is a theory called the three "R's", reassure, respond, and refocus. Using this approach, we can help them to feel safe and be their hero for the day or hour. Even though their beliefs are unfounded, they are very real to them.

I realize my loved one's paranoia is their reality at the time. I will reassure, respond, and refocus them to the best of my ability.

Emotional Honesty

Emotional honesty is taking responsibility for what we feel. It comes from recognizing and accepting what we feel rather than judging our feelings or blaming others. We all suffer from emotional pain at sometime or another. We feel that people do not understand our situation, or worse they do not care. The old saying "someone must be to blame if I am in pain" feeds into emotional self-destruction. Not being honest with ourselves about how we feel can lead to emotional destruction. Rather than focusing on what we can do to change the situation, we focus only on how bad it is. We may even feel unloved. The truth of the matter is that when we can fully accept who we are, we have taken the first step in healing our emotional wounds and ourselves.

I will be emotionally honest with myself so that I can feel whole and fulfilled.

Togetherness

We were a couple; we had a wonderful relationship. We were each other's best friend; in fact, we often finished each other's sentences. We had special moments together when we did not have to say a thing, and yet we knew what the other was thinking. These things are drifting away now that their disease is taking over. It is a sad situation. We may not be able to do all these things any longer, but no one can take the moments of the past away from us. They are part of who we were and who we are today. There can still be intimate times when our loved ones can show their love. A hug, a sweet smile or just having those quiet moments together are exchanges of affection that will be available even far into their disease process. If we embrace them, we can hold on to them forever.

*I will embrace our tender moments and
hold on to them forever.*

Distractions

An ordinary day can be filled with distractions for a person with dementia. They can have a difficult time staying in the moment. These distractions can make the simplest tasks difficult. It is hard to dress someone when they are moving around or distracted. The ringing of the phone, or watching TV while eating dinner, can push them completely off track. Our lives are also filled with distractions, but we are able to filter through them. Our loved one, on the other hand, has lost the ability to do this. When we are speaking to them, we should try to do so somewhere free of distractions. Turning off the TV and radio and making sure others are not having conversations in the same space will help. Through careful observation, we should be able to recognize things that distract them. We can then make a plan or redirect them in these difficult moments.

I will work to remove distractions from my loved one's life in hopes of making their life a little easier.

Burdens

We can place tremendous burdens on ourselves. We can be our own worst enemy. We believe that we need to get everything done today, and we should do it faster and better. We literally sabotage ourselves before we even get started. So what is the worst thing that can happen if we don't accomplish all we want to do today? Are the "caregiver police" going to arrest us? It is difficult to accomplish things when we feel burdened. The more pressure we place upon ourselves, the less likely we are to succeed. We do not need to prove anything to others. We do not have to answer to anyone but our higher power. We do not have to be a martyr or a superhero. We are doing the best we can and that is enough.

*I will stop looking at my perceived burdens
and change them into blessings.*

Sabotage

What is it about our personal nature that lets us sabotage ourselves? Is there a secret pay-off that we get from doing it? When we revert to old habits, or stop trying to accomplish a goal, it could be that little negative voice that keeps getting in our way. Self-Sabotaging behavior starts an internal tug-of-war. We think, "I never could have done that anyway, or I knew it was too good to be true". When we are self destructive, we lose faith in ourselves and give up. If we are going to overcome this self-sabotage, we first need to recognize it and confront it. We are stronger than we think, and self-defeating actions do not have to be part of our lives. If we slip up in our quest for a goal, it is o.k. We can start over again, only this time we have a little more knowledge to make it happen. We have learned from our past mistakes.

I will stop my self-destructive behavior and
work in a positive manner.

Far Away

Usually the person who lives the farthest away has the most to say. Our loved one is not as bad as we tell them they are; after all, since they have talked to them every month for two or three minutes, they should know. When someone offends us, our anger can make us defensive and can distort our line of reasoning. When this happens, we need to ask ourselves questions. Are they in denial about the severity of the disease? Do they feel guilty about living too far away? We also need to remember it is not about who is right or wrong, it is about meeting the needs of our loved one. Sometime the solution can be as easy as having them care for our loved one for a day or two. The picture will be much clearer to them when they have first-hand experience and "walk a mile in our shoes".

I will give my critics the opportunity to care for
my loved one so that they can have a clearer picture
of our every day problems.

Normal Aging

Dementia and Alzheimer's are not a normal part of aging. We know this now that our loved one has been diagnosed. However, most people do not know this. We have a special task that we now need to do, and that is to let others know the difference. Aging is hard enough without having severe memory loss added to it. Alzheimer's and dementia are more than a "senior moment". We need to share what we have learned about this disease so that others can make a timelier diagnosis if their loved ones are also stricken. This did not matter 10 year ago because we did not have any way to treat it. However, there are now medications to help slow the disease process down. Everyone wants to hedge their bet, and by sharing our knowledge, we can help them do that.

I will share my knowledge about this disease in hopes that I can ease someone's suffering.

May

∽

"We are shaped by our thoughts; we become what we think. When the mind is pure, joy follows like a shadow that never leaves."

BUDDHA QUOTE

Positive Self-Talk

Positive self-talk is the internal dialog we use to give ourselves positive reinforcements and self-motivation. We praise ourselves just as we would a friend. If we take away the negative and replace it with the positive, we can direct ourselves toward a better way of living our lives. Our minds learn from repetition so if we us positive self-talk and repeat them, eventually they will become part of who we are. If we repeatedly use positive self-talk we can recognize and act on our strengths. We can become more positive, more hopeful, and more effective. Such a mind-set will comfort us when things go wrong and affirm our positive attributes. Positive self-talk empowers us to handle our life with confidence and change our behavior as well as our thinking. It dictates the decisions we make, the actions we take, and the results we get.

I will practice positive self-talk and remove the negativity from my thoughts.

May 2

Adult Children

Even if our children live near by, we really do not want to bother them. They have lives of their own. They are busy with their jobs and children. We do not want to intrude on their lifestyle. If we continue to make excuses as to why we do not ask them to help, they may never know that they are needed. The fact is our children probably do want to help, but they just do not know how. Opening a dialogue with our children and asking for help is a positive action that can improve our communication with them. Adult children have said, they thought everything was good with their parents, and they did not know they even needed help. By giving them the opportunity to help, we are also teaching our grandchildren how to treat their parents, in the future. Children mimic what the see.

*I will speak with my children and let them
know how they can help.*

Attitude

Our attitude reflects how we see and react to all situations. If our glass is half-empty all the time, we cannot maintain balance in our lives. If we feel that our job as a caregiver is not fair and there is no way we can be happy in this role, our daily lives will be filled with discontent and anger. We need to remember that attitude is a choice. We cannot blame circumstances or other people for our negative attitude. The way we chose to see our lives is strictly up to us. How we respond to life's difficulties can say a great deal about our attitude. When we see life as good, we can then move forward and take positive action that leads us to positive solutions. We can turn obstacles into benefits. We are the ones that "make lemons into lemonade." Moreover, people enjoy being around other persons that have a positive outlook on life.

I will adjust my attitude and choose to have a great day.

Baggage

When we are going on a trip, we have to get our heavy luggage from point A to point B. In life, we also go from one destination to another, and we get caught up in this personal baggage. We all have this baggage, some of it comes from the outside, but most of it is self-imposed. It is a burden and it gets in our way. We even become defensive when others point it out to us. We rationalize and defend ourselves, but in the end, the baggage is still there and we continue to let it weigh us down. We need to take action to rid ourselves of this baggage so that we do not continue to stumble over it. First, we must take ownership of it and admit to ourselves that it is serving no positive function. We cannot change what we do not acknowledge. Life presents us with many obstacles, and it is our choice if we want to continue to trip over them or move forward.

I will begin to deal with my personal baggage so that I can free myself of its burden.

Independence

We all value our independence. We want to be self-sufficient; we want control over our lives. Persons with memory impairment want to retain their independence also. When it becomes necessary to limit certain activities, such as driving, cooking and other cognitive responsibilities, they will feel like we are being mean to them. It is usually safety-first issues, but because they are losing the ability to reason, they do not understand that. One of the most difficult things we have to do as caregivers is to tell our loved one that they can no longer do something. Things such as driving and cooking for themselves have been their ticket to independence. We may have to enlist the help of their doctor or the Department of Motor Vehicles when it comes to taking away their driving privileges. We can let them be the bad person. Whenever possible we need to let our loved one live as independent as they are capable of, but evaluating our loved one's capabilities is vital.

I will evaluate my loved one's capabilities and make sure they do not present a safety issue.

May 6

Lost

If our loved one wanders off and becomes lost, we are frantic with worry. We fear for their safety. We think about them being all alone and worry about how they are dressed. Will they be cold and get sick, or will they are overheated in the hot sun? All these thoughts and many more overwhelm us. This may be the scariest time we have ever encountered. To beat the odds we must be pro active. We need to register them with the Alzheimer's Associations, Safe Return Program. Today! Our local law enforcement agency needs to have all their pertinent information available on file. If they are getting out of the house, we need to put locks and alarm systems on all the doors. Neighbors need to be alerted to watch for them in case they get out alone. Doing what needs to be done ahead of time and having an action plan could make the difference between life and death.

I will become pro-active and attend to my loved ones safety immediately.

Limited Beliefs

Self-limiting beliefs are those things we believe about ourselves that place limitations on our abilities. They also create limited accomplishments and can deplete our energy. Our experiences form our beliefs. If we find that we have self-limited beliefs, it would serve us well to try to change them. For example, if we say, "I am not a good cook", we give ourselves an excuse not to cook. We do only what we believe we can do. Believing that we cannot achieve something, or letting our inner critic limit our actions, renders us powerless. Our beliefs have tremendous power over us. Once we identify our limiting beliefs, we can start the transformation to more positive ones. Changing our limited belief is a leap of faith and hard work but in the end, it is well worth it.

I will transform my limiting beliefs in to positive action.

Small Changes

Do we need to make radical changes in order to improve our lives? Probably not. Most of the time we only need to take the approach in baby steps. Small changes can make a big difference. Life is about change; we can choose to fight it, or embrace it. The outcome is directly related to how we handle the change. We need to recognize that our life is not a disaster, and by changing just a few things, we can make a difference. Our preconceived ideas can present obstacles to change. When we make changes, we want to see results and small changes allow us to do that. We need to remember never to ask anything of ourselves that we would not ask of others. When we give ourselves positive reinforcement, we will succeed in making small changes. With each accomplishment, we gain confidence in our ability to make these changes. Changes we choose reflect our ability to be flexible and give our life a welcome freshness.

I will embrace small changes and
welcome the positive results.

Wish

"I wish they would stop following me around all the time. I can barely go to the bathroom alone". Repetitive behavior is a common problem in Alzheimer's. It is important to know that our loved one is not trying to annoy us, nor are they doing this on purpose. We wish they would stop repeating and asking the same questions over and over again. There is nothing bad about these thoughts. It is normal to want annoying behavior to stop. Many times, they are just looking for reassurance that we are still there. Eventually, these things will stop, but usually not until they have had a decline. When the decline happens, they may not be able to walk well or express themselves clearly. Maybe their annoying behavior is not that bad after all. Some of God's greatest gifts are unanswered prayers ... Garth Brooks.

Even though my loved ones repetitive behavior bothers me, I will continue to reassure them of my love.

May 10

Normal

Some days our loved one can seem so normal that we forget they have memory problems. Although these days or moments are welcomed, we need to be careful not to overreact and expect too much from them. Our reasoning can be blurred, and these times can lead to false hope, even though we know they are not going to get better. When these types of days or moments present themselves, we should welcome them as a gift. If we hold them tightly and imprint them on our hearts, they will be there in the future to draw on. Good days are there to remind us that we are caring for a wonderful person that deserves our undying love. We need to be grateful for the good days. They are there to validate the good in our lives.

I will hold my loved one's good days tightly to my heart and welcome them as a gift.

In The Beginning

In the beginning, our loved one may or may not have been aware of their memory loss. They did however know that something was not right. The fear of having the "Big A" as some call it, is overwhelming. They may have denied that they had a problem. Meanwhile, frustration and depression began to set in. Being confused, they even blamed us for things that became lost or accuse us of trying to make them look bad. By now we have probably gone through this early part of the disease. Our loved one now is not aware that they cannot remember things, or that they are not communicating properly. If there is anything good to be said about the progression, it is that this is the beginning of the more merciful parts of the disease for them. If they were aware of what was going on with their minds and bodies, they would be devastated.

I will do everything in my power to help my loved one get through this disease with their dignity in tact.

Dentist

Are there really people out there that enjoy going to the dentist? Somehow, I don't think so. It is important for us to have regular dental check ups, and it may be even more important for our loved one to have regular check ups. For the most part, they cannot tell us when something hurts, or when they have lost a filling. Preventative medicine is the best choice. The selection of a dentist must be carefully considered. We first need to speak personally to the dentist, so that he knows the problem. By making plans with the dentist about procedures, possible behavior problems, and the use of sedation, the visit will be less traumatizing to all involved. Pain caused by dental problems is not an option, but the cost and extent of a procedure must be weighted with common sense. We are the final decision makers.

*I will seek a dentist that is knowledgeable
and compassionate towards my loved.*

Really Listening

Everyone likes to think that they are good listeners, but true listening is a skill, it takes practice. First, we need to stop that inner voice that is just waiting for a small pause in the conversation so that we can talk. If we are anticipating what we are going to say, we are not really listening. When we are mentally dissecting and judging what a person is saying, we are not listening, and we are not being kind. It is not our intention to be mean, but sometimes we are so busy making sure that people hear what we have to say that we forget to listen. It is not enough that we are listening to someone, but we want to let them know that we are listening and that they have our undivided attention. The art of listening is a wonderful gift that we can give to others and ourselves. When we listen to others, we show that what they have to say is worthwhile. People like to surround themselves with good listeners.

I will sharpen my listening skills so that I can
hear what others really have to say.

May 14

Understanding Behaviors

Before we can manage a behavior, we must first understand the cause. We need to examine the situation and try to find the source. Is our loved one in pain, over tired, hungry, or physically uncomfortable? Are we asking them to do something they are no longer capable of doing? Is their environment calm and familiar? These simple situations are often the keys managing a challenging behavior. We must remember that we set the tempo. When we are argumentative or angry with them, it can spill over and magnify their behavior. A good first step to managing these behaviors is to minimize confusion and anxiety, and to adapt our loved one's environment to their capabilities. No matter how much we love someone, we will at times become anxious or angry. Even though we know, we should be calm and patient, it is sometimes challenging for us to.

I will try to understand my loved one's problem behavior
patterns and help them through these times.

How Do You Do That

People often say to us, "I don't know how you accomplish all that you have to do." You know what? There are times when we do not know either. What we do know is that we are doing the best we can for the person we love. Sometimes we can see the pieces of the puzzle but do not know how to solve it. In the end, the pieces come together and the problem is solved. We do more than just put one foot in front of the other. We use our creativity to form the best possible environment for our loved one. We use our problem solving skills to make life simpler, and we use our sense of humor to lighten the load. We can do what we do because we believe in ourselves and know that all things are possible.

I believe in myself and will do whatever it takes to get through this journey.

May 16

Saying Goodbye

It's a long and sad road we must travel in saying goodbye to our loved one with Alzheimer's. There is a reason why it is called "the Long Goodbye". The person afflicted may take as many as 10 years to physically die. We watch them on this long journey, and each time they lose a function or the ability to do a simple task, we grieve. This "anticipatory grief" begins very early in this disease. We see the person that we have known and loved for years turn into a stranger. When we witness the slow death of their minds and loss of bodily functions, we begin to say goodbye, even though they are still with us physically. We are never ready for the end no matter how much we think we are. This Eskimo proverb may help us cope better with our grief: "Perhaps they are not stars, but rather openings in heaven, where the love of our lost ones pours through, and shines down upon us, to let us know they are happy."

If my grief becomes too strong, I will seek help so that I can be there for my loved one.

Laughter

Laughter does more than make us feel good. It helps us release some of our pent-up emotions. It also helps us put things in perspective. "Maybe things are not as bad as we think." Laughter helps bring balance into our life. Our life is not all gloom and doom. Remember laughter is contagious, and it could spread to those we care for. Doctor Patch Adams of the Gesundheit Institute (yes like in sneeze) believes that laughter, joy and creativity are an integral part of healing. He believes that "you can treat a disease and you may win or you can treat a person and you will always win". We all need a laugh sometime. Even Mark Twain had the vision of laughter in medicine, and he said it well, "Against the assaults of laughter nothing can stand". So is laughter the best medicine? It would appear that it is.

In an effort to lift my spirits and those of my loved one, I will remember that laughter can be the best medicine.

Respect

Even though our loved one may act like a child and demonstrate childlike behavior, this does not give us the right to treat them like a child. As the disease progress, their demeanor begins to decline, and they exhibit a lack of impulse control. It is difficult to see our loved one in this childish state and not react negatively, but when we over react to their behavior, it will just escalate. If they could see themselves in this behavioral state, they would be humiliated and sad. The best action at these times is no reaction. If we become argumentive or try to correct them, we will only make the problem worse. Redirecting is always a good choice at these times. Not only do we need to respect them for the person they are, but also we must insist that others treat them the same. Overlooking their child like behavior will make everyone's day more enjoyable.

I will overlook my loved ones child like behavior and remember it is not them, it is the disease.

Feeling Good

When was the last time we really felt good about ourselves? If we cannot remember that moment, we need to take a personal inventory. What is it about our lives that block those feelings? Are we so full of negativity that we do not recognize the loving, caring person we are? Feeling good about who we are and what we do, sets the standard for how we want others to treat us. We should never judge our skills and self worth against that of others. By recognizing our self-worth, we can then move forward and reinforce our positive thoughts. It is much easier to perform a task or stay in our social circle when we feel good about ourselves. Our love for ourselves should come first; when it does, we are then prepared to share it with others.

I will take a personal inventory and do what ever it takes so that I can feel good about myself.

A Shoulder to Cry On

Sometimes we just need a shoulder to cry on. We need someone to listen, someone who will understand what our days are like, someone who is walking the same journey. We cannot always depend on a family member to be there for us. They may not know the full extent of our caregiver responsibilities. Being able to express ourselves and just say how we feel would be an incredible relief. These are just a few of the benefits we can receive by joining a support group. We want to be surrounded by people who can relate to us. Being able to speak freely to people who are going, or have gone through some of the same thing as us can prove to be one of the best supportive actions we can take. We also will have the opportunity to learn how others cope and make new friends at the same time. It is a win-win situation for everyone.

I will look for a support group to attend so that I will have a sounding board for my problems.

Self Doubt

All caregivers suffer from self-doubt at sometime during their journey of care. Unfortunately, when we try to discuss this with others, such as friends or even family, we may hear, "I don't know how you do it, or I just couldn't stand it," or "why don't you just put them in a nursing home". When we hear these things, we are thrown off balance. Just when we thought we were doing   pretty well, someone throws us a curve, and we begin to doubt our abilities and our decisions. The important thing we need to remember is not to let self-doubt stop us from succeeding. It is said that if we doubt ourselves we usually end up talking ourselves out of success. We are doing a good. job. No, a great job. Christian Bovee said, "Doubt whom you will, but never yourself". If we are harboring doubt, we need repeat this phrase over and over until we believe it.

I am doing a great job. This will be my mantra for the day.

May 22

Hold On

There may be times when just holding on is all we can do. We are tired, our loved one is going through a challenging time, and our life seems to have come to a halt. Hold on. Yes holding on is all we really need to do right now. We need to take a personal adult time out. We only need to do what has to be done right now. Surprisingly enough, our house will not crumble around us, and our life will be just fine. We tend to push ourselves too hard at times. Our goals may be unrealistic, thus we become frustrated and do not know where to turn. If we continue at this fast pace, we could succumb to health problems caused by stress. Our mind and body know it is time to slow down, and it is giving us a warning that we need to heed.

I will heed the warning of my body and take things more slowly so that I will not succumb to stress.

Gift of Guilt

Truly, guilt is "The "Gift" that keeps on Giving". Unfortunately, it is almost an inescapable reality for caregivers. Things go wrong, and we play the "would a, should a, if only" blame game. The self-imposed standards we place on ourselves are not realistic. We ask more of ourselves than we do of others. Our unspoken feelings of guilt continue to grow. Part of our solution to freeing ourselves of guilt is to take ownership. We need to acknowledge it before we can work through it. By setting realistic goals and stopping our inner negative talk, we can see more clearly and move forward for a solution. Sometimes there are no straightforward answers, and the best we can do is ask for forgiveness. By forgiving ourselves of our past transgressions, we become stronger and no longer need to be stuck in the guilt trap.

I will not accept the "gift" of guilt. I will forgive myself and move forward in my life.

May 24

Why

We often ask the question why. When we ask the "Why Question" of someone with dementia, it will only lead to frustration and confusion. They do not know why they did or did not do something. As their capacity to reason diminishes, they cannot comprehend why. By asking why, we are heading towards confrontation causing them to become defensive or angry. Most forms of questions will be difficult for them to answer because it involves a searching process of the mind, and they are no longer able to perform this search. We should never argue or try to change their minds when they become confrontational; instead, we need to practice patient communication. Remember, it is more confusing for them then it is for us. We should just move on in our communication. Supportive care is essential to their well-being. Just because they are stuck does not mean we have to be.

I will refrain from asking questions of my loved one and try to communicate more effectively.

Finances

Money is one of the last things we want to talk about when we are caring for someone with Alzheimer's. Unfortunately, it needs to be one of the first things we deal with. Unlike other diseases, we have a limited time to address this issue. As their memories fail and their cognitive skills decline, our window of opportunity is closing. In an ideal world, it is best to work as a family unit, but in the real world that is not always possible. There are so many facets of finances that need to be addressed that it may benefit us to work with a professional. It is not worth having hard feelings among family members, especially in these difficult times. The old axiom, "money is the root of all evil" can be true in many instances, so it is our responsibility to approach the topic with candor.

I will try to work through the financial maze, and if I have problems, I will enlist the help of a professional.

Rest and Replenish

Professional athletes rest between games. People in very warm climates take siestas. These types of rest are considered a necessity rather than a luxury. Resting and replenishing can be done in many ways meditation, reading, yoga, physical exercise, or massage. The problem is that most of us do not know how to allow our body and mind to rest during the daytime. Little wonders that depression, and exhaustion plagues us caregivers. There are many ways to replenish our energy but taking a physical rest is probably the best for most people. Napping for a brief period can be pleasurable and it gives the mind and body a break. We do not have to fall into a deep sleep in order to replenish. Our needs always seem to come last but we cannot keep giving if we do not take time to replenish ourselves. Just closing our eyes: even for a brief rest has the benefit of reducing stress and it can give us more energy while improving our cognitive function.

I will try to rest for a short time each day so that
I can function better all day long.

Dual Jobs

Sometimes caregiving is a dual job. We find ourselves doing a balancing act. Our children, husband, wife, grandchildren need our attention. We are the true sandwich generation. Being the perpetual caregiver we are, we want to take care of everyone, when in truth we are having a hard time being the primary caregiver for our loved one. Our normal lifestyle as we knew it is changing. We do not have time to do the things we enjoy like being with our grand children or children. Our days are filled with things that we must do in order to keep our loved one safe and happy. In order to alleviate the strain we feel, we must know our limits how much can we do, and how far can we go with out crashing. If we stretch ourselves too far, there will be no winner. This balancing act can only succeed if we invite others to help.

I will come to terms with my limits, and not overstep them.
I will ask for help when I need it.

Trust Our Inner Voice

One of our main sources of wisdom comes from our inner voice. It can be like a premonition, intuition, or just a gut feeling. It is a feeling or sensation that wants our attention. Sometimes we feel silly listening to our inner voice because we cannot prove it is there. We are, however, familiar with our inner voice because in the past it may have prompted us to do something that we did not follow through on. After the fact we thought, "I should have followed my gut feeling and listened to myself". Our inner voice really is the essence of who we are and what we do. It is a signal that warns us of danger or tells us to rethink a problem. If we have faith in our inner voice and connect with our inner most feelings, we will have a wonderful sense of self-acceptance.

I will trust my inner voice and use its guidance to help solve my everyday problems.

Body Language

We have all heard the saying, "actions speak louder than words". However, it has never meant more than now when we are trying to communicate with someone that is memory impaired. As our loved one's ability to process verbal information declines, we may need to use body language even more. Statistically as much as 90 per cent of our communication takes place through non-verbal communication such as gestures, facial expressions, and touch. The way we hold our arms, folded and crossed close to our body, says "I am mad or impatient". When talking to our loved one our facial expressions can mean more than our words. They can respond to our body language long after their ability to understand our words is gone. We must be mindful of how we look when we speak. Even if we are angry or mad, we should never show it.

I will keep my body language positive and be mindful of the impact it has on my loved one.

Hopeful

Being hopeful is positive thinking in action. Hope is a feeling of desire and fulfillment. Martin Luther tells us "We must accept finite disappointment, but we must never lose infinite hope". When we view our life with hope, we become optimistic and our self-esteem is boosted. Our hopefulness enhances our ability to conquer our hardships and overcome extreme challenges. Hope should not be a fleeting thought, but instead be our constant companion. Hopeful people make things happen for the better. Our optimistic thinking helps us see the positive in our lives. Having hope is being sure that what we do today will have a positive effect in the lives of others. Doom and Gloom do not belong in our life. Hope allows us to see the rainbow, even if it rains on our parade.

I will welcome hope as my constant companion and use it to guide me.

Clinging

One thing that can drive us crazy is when our loved one constantly clings to us, or follows us wherever we go, even to the bathroom. This probably ranks in the top 10 problems caregivers experience. Because their memory impairment impedes their sense of timing, they panic if they cannot see us. When we leave the room, they do not know that we are not leaving them and we will be back. This behavior may be more prevalent towards evening. It is referred to as "Sundowning" a term used to describe the increased confusion and agitation that occurs later in the day and evening. We are their security blanket we make. We make them feel safe. We can try to redirect them or give them something to do. Again, by being creative in our approach, we may be able to get a temporary fix. This phase does not go on forever so learning to deal with it may be the best approach.

I will not get upset when my loved one clings to
me for I am their safety net in life.

June

∽

"Each player must accept the cards life deals him or her: but once they are in hand, he or she alone must decide how to play the cards in order to win the game."

VOLTAIRE

Golden Years

We all look towards our golden years as a time to travel and do the thing we never had time to do before. Unfortunately, the golden years become tarnished as this disease consumes our loved one. The thought of leaving our loved one at home, as we go out and enjoy ourselves, fill us with grief and guilt. It was not our plan to go out and enjoy our leisure time by ourselves. Now we feel guilty if we pursue these pleasures so we deprive ourselves of enjoying them and we become isolated. Being a victim does not benefit anyone; in fact, it makes us more unapproachable. The truth is that it is OK to pursue the thing we love, as long as our loved one is safe and well cared for. Being a martyr will serve no purpose and make us feel resentful towards our loved one.

I will begin to pursue the things I love and not feel guilty when I enjoy them.

June 2

Replenish

We were taught from a very young age not to waste time. We needed to keep busy if we were going to be productive people. "Idle hands are the devils workshop" and all that stuff. This is a lesson we need to reevaluate. Our bodies physically and emotionally need some down time to relax. We cannot replenish if we do not take the time to refuel. If we cannot remember the last time we relaxed in a nice warm bath, then it has been too long. We are so busy meeting other's needs that we fail to recognize our own. Unstructured activities like enjoying the sunset or taking that nice warm bubble bath are great antidotes for stress. We cannot give what we do not have. We need to be as diligent about refreshing and replenishing our bodies as we are about caring for our loved one.

I will make time to relax and enjoy the
things that make me happy.

Believe

If there was ever a time in our lives when we need to believe in ourselves, it is now. We need to believe that we are doing the best we can. By believing in ourselves, we are empowered to recognize our needs and those of our loved one, with out feeling guilty. We need to take pride in our accomplishments. Caregiving takes courage and if we do not believe in ourselves, we cannot expect other to do so. Each day brings new challenges that we can deal with if we trust our caregiving skills and ourselves. When we believe in ourselves, we will have a positive self-image. The actions we take and the effort we make, are a direct reflection of what we believe. Our own self-belief will help us succeed in all we do. When we embrace who and what we are, our achievements are unlimited.

I will take pride in what I do and
applaud my accomplishments.

June 4

Tube Feeding

In the later stages of Alzheimer's, chewing and swallowing can become difficult and in many cases, they can no longer swallow without choking. Artificial nutrition such as tube feeding is a controversial and an emotional issue that many caregivers may have to face. Hopefully, our loved one's wishes are in place, in a living will, but even then this may be the hardest decision we will ever have to make. Our biggest fear may be that we are letting them die by starving them to death. It is believed by much of the medical community that in the last stages of dementia, a person's organs shut down, and they do not feel hunger. However, there is no proof of that. The best thing we can do when faced with this dilemma is to ask ourselves, who's needs am I thinking of, theirs or mine. There is no one answer to the feeding tube dilemma.

If the feeding tube dilemma arises, I will make the most compassionate decision I can make.

Humor in Everyday Life

Humor is a personal ability to evoke amusement, laughter, or happiness in themselves or others. Sometimes the best way to handle tension or stress is through humor. I could have laughed or cried. I chose to laugh. In our world of everyday caregiving many things happen that are just plain funny. It is ok to see humor in our lives as long as it is not at the expense of others. It allows us to see things in a different perspective, and it helps us to see beyond out hardships. Humor is a gift that helps us see, that life goes on. The humor we find in tragedy makes it tolerable. Appropriate uses of humor can help us feel that life is worth living fully. You cannot hold tension and laugh at the same time. Mark Twain said it well "the secret source of humor is not joy, but sorrow.

I will look for the humor in even the
most difficult situations.

Tender Moments

If we have known love then, we have known tender moments. These moments have brought us warmth and joy in the past. We wonder if we will ever experience these feelings again now that we are immersed in our role of caregiver. Now more than ever, our life is all about love. The only way we can do this is out of love and compassion. These moments can be as simple as their sweet smile, shared laughter, or a simple look of recognition when they seem the most lost. If we share these tender moments of laughter, tears, and compassion, we will never become the victim. What we have gained from our caregiving experience far outweighs what we have given. John Ruskin speaks about what a person gets for their toil: "The highest reward for a person's toil is not what they get for it, but what they become by it."

*I will value the tender moments so that I can
draw on them in my time of need.*

Friends

Friendship can be one of the most valued assets of life. Friendships need to be nurtured. Just because we are caregiving is no reason to abandon our friends. Friendships that we have nurtured throughout our lives are even more important now. One way to foster our friendship is to show that we appreciate our friends. Our friends want to assist us but do not know what we need. Sometimes they do not know how to help simply because we have not asked them to. No job is too big or small for a true friend. If we suggest specific things that we need assistance with it will help our friends know how to help us. "A friend is someone who understands your past, believes in your future, and accepts you just the way you are." In Mister Rogers's neighborhood, he says, "You don't have to be anything more than what you are right now", and true friends know that.

I will nurture my friendships and show them
appreciation for standing by me.

June 8

Insecurity

Our insecurities stop us from feeling comfortable with ourselves. It causes us to question our judgment and abilities. Insecurity is an invasion of negative thoughts and feelings. In essence, we play tug-of-war with ourselves and give into our fears. We worry about being good enough and feel like we have to prove something. We want to have the love and admiration of others. These feeling are uncomfortable and need to stop. Using our inner resources, we can move forward with confidence and reinstate our self-esteem. Knowing all the good we do is one thing, believing in all the good we do is another. Breaking the barrier of self-doubt allows us to let go of the past and move on. It does not really matter where our insecurity comes from. It only matters what we do with and about it.

I will review all the good that I do
and be secure in all that I do.

Share the Wisdom

We can recall the day we were told our loved one had Alzheimer's. Life is unpredictable, but we certainly did not expect to have anyone we know and love to be diagnosed with this disease. Looking back, we know what it felt like to be scared and to feel alone. We may have thought that no one could possibly understand what we are going through and we did not know how we were going to make it. Hopefully there came a time when we realized that we were not alone. Time also gave us the strength to get through each day. We learned that our love and strength are stronger than we ever dreamed they could be. We do not have to be experts in order to share our knowledge and wisdom. Drawing on our experiences, we can now share our wisdom with others who are just starting their journey.

I will share my wisdom and knowledge of this disease with others that are just beginning their journey.

Grump Days

We all have grump days, when even our very best just does not seem good enough. On grump days, we cannot seem to get it together. Yes, everyone has them or they would not be human in fact, some people even set aside a special day and designate it "Grump Day". When we are having a good old grump day, we do not need to feel bad about having it. It is our right to be grumpy as long as we do not impose it on anyone else. When this day comes we cannot just take the day off and go back to bed, but we can take the day off, sort of. We need to set everything aside and only do what is necessary. If we are brave enough to take this day for ourselves, we will be rewarded with renewed energy and attitude. Remember, it was Grumpy who lead the charge to save Snow White from the Wicked Queen.

I will take the day off the next time I have a grump day and not feel guilty about doing it.

Delegating

Caregivers are not known for their ability to delegate. We want control, and it is hard to trust others to do parts of our jobs. We are sure that others cannot do them as well. We work so hard to make things right for our loved one that giving up any of the control to someone else is difficult. We have been so focused on being self sufficient that we have lost sight of our goal. Eventually we need to trust others. Surrendering is not giving up our power; it is enhancing it with the assistance of others. There are times when we need to surrender to the situation. Giving up some of our control can be scary, but we need to recognize that we cannot do everything ourselves. It is so easy for us to help others, but taking other's help is foreign to us.

I will trust others and begin to delegate
so that I can lighten my load.

June 12

Miracles Around Us

Miracles are not just supernatural events that happen to everyone else. They are happening around us every day. The word miracle means "something wonderful". Miracles are the random events that give meaning to our life. Receiving a phone call from someone we love, when at the time, we were feeling unloved. The near miss of a car accident is often called a miracle. We do not need an explanation for everything some things are unexplainable. How could we possibly explain a spider web or the emerging of a butterfly from a cocoon? There are thousands of miracles around us everyday. S.Parkes Cadman asks; "What is more supernatural than an egg yoke turning into a chicken?" A rainbow after a storm is truly extraordinary. Call them what we will they are miraculous acts. We too perform miracles, every time we reach out and help someone. There are miracles in our sharing, our compassion; and especially, in our acts of love!

I will carefully look around me for the miracles of life.

Working with Our Doctor

Together with our doctor, we need to make a plan of care for our loved one. We ask how that is possible since he is only in the room such a short time. It is our duty to make sure all of our questions are answered. We can do this by being explicit when answering or asking a question. Most importantly, we need to speak up and continue to ask the question until we understand completely. By preparing for the visit ahead of time, we will come away more satisfied. Making list of problems is always a good plan of action. Include things such as a change in behavior; our loved one suddenly cannot sleep through the night, or they have started to be incontinent. A list of all medications even over the counter medicines need to be given in written form to the doctor or nurse so that it will become part of our loved one's records. If we can schedule some time alone with the doctor we are on the road to good health care.

*I will work with my doctor to assure my loved
one gets the best health care possible.*

June 14

Tell Someone

How and when we tell someone about our loved one's disease is a personal preference. For the good of our loved one and ourselves, we eventually need to share this information with others. They probably already know something is wrong, but they do not know what it is or how bad it is. Shouldering this responsibility alone can be overwhelming. If we look at a disease as having a stigma attached, we put up roadblocks for understanding and help. People cannot understand the hardship or burden we carry if we do not talk to them about it. By sharing this information, we give them the opportunity to understand and offer their support in whatever form they can. Problems do not seem so big when shared. If we are open with this information, we give people a better sense of what is happening in our life and how they can assist us.

I will be open and honest about my loved one's diagnosis, and give people the opportunity to assist me.

Sacrifice

When we take responsibility for someone else, it usually involves some personal sacrifice. As a caregiver, we are making concessions a lot of the time. It does not matter if the sacrifice is big or small; we are dealing with life changing decisions. We do not often think of what we do as sacrifice, because we are doing it out of love and compassion. We want the very best for our loved one and we are willing to go the extra mile to get it. Self-sacrifice for someone else is a sign of character and strength. It is also an act of generosity and love. We do not expect to be repaid for what we do; in fact, we would be insulted if someone tried. Through sacrifice, we find meaning in our own lives. Self-sacrifice is one of the highest forms of love and care. Done willingly and of free spirit everyone will win.

I will use my sacrifices as the highest form
of love for my loved one.

Why Me

If we ask "why me God" then we have to answer "why not me" God is not singling us out or punishing us. Being a person that wants to be in control, we want to understand and know why. We often think that because we are a good person that this should not have happened. We become confused when bad things happen and ask God why. What was God thinking of anyway? What we are really asking is for the pain to go away. There is a bumper sticker that says S### happens, and it sometimes does. We can look for the answer all we want, but the answer is, "it just is." If we can let go of the "why", we can begin to take control of our lives and learn to manage and live each day with quality. It is said that we have no right to ask when a sorrow comes, "Why did this happen to me?" unless we ask the same question for every joy that comes our way."

I will stop questioning why this happened and concentrate on living the best life possible.

Teachers

Life brings us many teachers. We may not view them as teachers because they are the people we see and work with every day. Life's teachers do not have to be in a classroom. Friends in support groups may teach us a new technique or coping skill. Our church or synagogue can teach us tolerance and forgiveness. If we look back at a favorite teacher we had in school, we will see that they were the ones that challenged us the most. Life's lessons are not always fair or kind, but if we learn from them, we will become stronger and more confident in all that we do. If we pay attention to the people around us, we just may learn something when we least expect it. Experiences of life are great teachers.

I will pay attention to life's teachings and learn from them.

Life's Purpose

The most basic questions everyone faces in life are, "why am I here?" or "What is my purpose?" We sometimes wake up in the morning and think, "is this all there is?" Caregiving can drain us physically and mentally. We know what our job is, but what is our purpose in the grand scheme of things? We are not defined by the job of caregiving. If we take some time to look at all we have accomplished in our lives, we would be overwhelmed. We may not be able to stand up and state our purpose, but we are making a difference every day. The author Robert Byrne sums it up for us, "the purpose of life is a life of purpose." We can read one of the many books that talk about life and purpose but the testament of purpose is the action we take in our life. We have accomplished much, and should be proud.

I will live my life with purpose and be proud
of what I have accomplished.

Magic Window

If we had a magic window where we could see and hear into the heart and soul of our loved one, what would we see and hear? They might be saying, "even though my actions don't reflect the person I was, please treat me as such". There is still a person in here and I love you. Don't hurry me. Each day it's a struggle to keep up. Be patient with me, my brain is what causes me to sometimes be out of control. Thank you for taking such good care of me. I wish I could take some of your burden away. Sometimes I am afraid, but you make me feel safe. Pray for me, for I am drifting between time and reality. Laugh with me I still have a sense of humor. Be compassionate with me. Hold me and touch me with your loving hands. I feel loved when you do. Most of all, love me with all your heart and soul. You are my guardian angel on earth."

I will open my heart and love my loved one unconditionally.

Judgmental

Family and friends can be judgmental at times. They think we are exaggerating our loved one's condition. They may make a comment when we finally take some personal time away from our loved one. They may disapprove of us placing our loved one in day care or a nursing facility. When we think that we are being judged, we can lose our temper and lash out. On the other side of our feelings, we may cave in and try to please them, even if we do not think they are right. At other times, we act like there is nothing wrong, and we stuff our feelings. It is at this time our emotional pressure builds, and we become overly stressed. It is possible that they will never change their minds. They can never walk in our shoes, and we pray they do not have to. Someday they may understand, but until then we should not sit in judgment of them. Our best defense is compassion and forgiveness.

I will not judge those who judge me. I will show them compassion and forgiveness.

Preparedness

We must prepare for death as we have prepared for life, no matter how uncomfortable it makes us. Our families must know what kind of treatment we want if we are terminally ill. They need to know what we want done after we die. Not only do we need to talk about this with our families, but we also need to have it in writing. The documents we need to complete are called advance directives. They include a living will and durable power of attorney for health care. What do we want our families to do if we are deemed terminal or cannot make health care decisions ourselves. How do we want to spend our last days? What comfort measures do we want? Who do we want to make these decisions for us when we can't? We need to spell it out so that when the time comes our families can fulfill our wishes and be comfortable in doing so.

*I will begin to take action on the legal documents
that will direct my final days.*

June 22

Wisdom

Wisdom comes with the experience of age. It is acquired not learned. Our everyday experiences make us wiser. Wisdom compels us to listen before we act. Sometimes we gain a deeper appreciation of wisdom because of making mistakes and learning from them. The wisdom we gain allows us to make informed choices, and good decisions. Wisdom offers us guidance and understanding of the important things in life. Wisdom is the application of knowledge. It is gained by observing life and learning from the failures and successes of others and ourselves. In caregiving, we can gain wisdom from other caregivers and look toward professionals for added wisdom. If we use the resources available to us and ask question of those in the know, wisdom can be our tool of self-growth. Wisdom gives us direction and acts as a compass that guides us through life.

I will rely on wisdom to guide me through life.

Count Our Blessings

By counting our blessings, we have the opportunity to enjoy the little things in life. We need to be thankful for the good and the bad. We can be fulfilled despite our set backs. When we are grateful, we can find fulfillment in all that we do. There are times when we take the good things for granted. We have a multitude of things to be thankful for and yet if asked to recite them we might hesitate for a minute. If we were to take a piece of paper and write down the things we are thankful for, we may start slow, but we will pick up momentum and our list will grow long. By forgetting our woes, we will be able to focus on the blessings that are bestowed upon us daily. Unity co-founder Charles Fillmore wrote, "It has been found by experience that a person increases his blessings by being grateful for what he has."

I will count my blessings and be thankful for what I have.

Relaxation

The everyday stress of caring for our loved one will manifest itself in many ways. We may not sleep well, over eat, or drink, all in the name of reducing stress. These ways of dealing with stress will only make us more stressed. There are many ways to achieve relaxation, none of which include over indulging. We need to be willing to make life changes by starting to change the way we react to stressful situations in our daily lives. Although we can all benefit from relaxation, most of us either do not know how to relax, or feel we just do not have the time. If we give ourselves permission to let go and relax, we have taken the first step in renewing our spirit and body. No one technique of relaxing is right for everyone. We need to explore the right one that fits our life style. Relaxation will help us achieve inner calm and a more balanced life.

I will learn to relax, so that I can better manage my stress.

Gratefulness

We all have many things to be grateful for but sometimes we focus on the thing we do not have. In our haste to accomplish things, we forget to be thankful. When we focus on what we are grateful for, we are reminded of our priorities and what is important to us. It is the simple thing in life that gives us pleasure. Our home, our children, pets, and friends are vitally important. Our lives are filled with beauty if only we take the time to claim it. If we take the time to really look at our life, we will realize we have much to be grateful for. When we are grateful, we are happier and more content. Gratitude begets gratitude and attract good thing in our lives. The more we feel grateful the more we will attract thing to be grateful for. Gratitude is an attribute we should all strive to attain.

I will look at my life and be grateful for all that I have.

June 26

There is a Season

Some of the most quoted words of the Bible are, "to everything there is a season, a time for every purpose under the sun". Our life is in a constant process of change. There is no way to stop it, so it is best to go with the flow. Even though we do not always understand it, we should recognize that it does have a purpose. Change at times can present a challenge, but there is always light at the end of the tunnel. It may take us time to find it, but it is there. We have learned to navigate the challenges in life and transitions have become smoother. From every beginning, there is an end, and that may be the hardest thing in life to accept, even though it is inevitable. We need to trust that when something ends, something else will begin. We should not fear the flow of change; instead, we need to learn to embrace it.

I will take comfort in knowing that everything has a season, and when something ends, something else will follow.

Patience

We all struggle from time to time with being patient. It is especially difficult to be patient with our loved one when they repeat the same thing over and over. When they are unable to perform a simple task, we become frustrated and often impatient. We lose our patience and become angry. The more frustrated we get, the more the problem feeds upon itself and takes on a life of its own. Being patient, even in the fast pace world we live in, is indeed a virtue that we all need to practice. Throwing in the towel is not an option. There is a Chinese Proverb that says it all: "If you are patient in one moment of anger, you will escape a hundred days of sorrow". If we can mentally step back and quiet our mind, we may be able to escape those days of sorrow.

I will practice patience in all that I do.

Doing My Best

If there was ever a mantra we should all recite it is "I am doing my best." We become so busy caregiving that when things are going smoothly, we forget that we are the ones that made it happen. It is easy to beat up on ourselves, but difficult to give ourselves the proverbial pat on the back. Remember, we do not have a "how to book" of caregiving, and we did not have anyone train us in this newfound job. We dash from one commitment to another without even acknowledging all the good that we do. If we continue to ignore the good we do, we will create a life of discontent. This is not being egotistical or pompous; it is simply recognizing our self worth. We can stand tall for we are doing an outstanding job.

I will repeat to myself "I am doing the best I can" and stop criticizing myself when things go wrong.

Be All That We Can Be

The army slogan say: "be all that you can be." How does that pertain to us and what exactly does it mean? We can break it down simply. It is doing our best while being true to ourselves. It also means going the extra mile and most importantly knowing how to let go. Over time not living in accordance with our true self, takes a tremendous toll. Letting go of anger and resentment will free us to be all that we can be. It will decrease our negativity and increase our self-esteem. We also need to know our limits, because they are a strong part of what and who we are. Knowing who we are and what we are capable of lets our self-confidence show through. Positive attracts positive and people will feel comfortable around us. Every thing that we put into ourselves benefit all those around us.

*I will strive to be all that I can be while
keeping my limitations in focus.*

June 30

Hearing the Diagnosis

We probably knew the truth long before we were ready to admit it. We had our suspicions and knew something was wrong long before we were given the diagnosis. We weren't being neglectful. It was just too bitter a pill to swallow. It was an extremely difficult time for us and our loved one. Indirectly we thought that if we didn't go to the doctors and hear the diagnosis it was not true; it would just go away. We even thought that once it was given a name "Alzheimer's," life as we knew it would be over. In retrospect we were so filled with fear that we already had stopped enjoying life. We were afraid of what others would think of our loved one. We were afraid that we wouldn't be able to care for them. A big part of the fear is the uncertainty and the feeling that we have lost control of our life. We do not need to be afraid anymore. We have stepped up and have taken control.

I will not fear the unknown, but will meet it
head on with my courage and fortitude.

July

∽

Too often we underestimate the power of a touch, a smile, a kind word, a listening ear, an honest compliment, or the smallest act of caring, all of which have the potential to turn a life around.

LEO F. BUSCAGLIA

Positive Affirmations

Affirmation means, "To make firm". By using affirmations in our daily lives, we can teach the conscious mind to act in a positive manner. Positive self-talk is similar to visualization because they help create positive images. They work best when they are short sentences or a series of words. We need to make them believable and achievable. They should always be personal and about us. They can be most helpful if spoken when negative thoughts begin to invade our space. There is a theory that "like attracts like." Simply said, we attract into our life what we think about. Positive affirmations used frequently throughout the day will help us rise above the negative self-talk we speak to ourselves. They guide our thoughts away from the negative. We should try to use them frequently throughout the day. They are a positive way to start the day and a good way to settle ourselves in for the evening. There is no right or wrong place to do them. The key is doing them.

I will begin and end my days with positive affirmations and rise above any negative talk.

July 2

Challenges

Though out our life we face many challenges, most of which we are able to overcome. Now that we are faced with caregiving for someone with memory loss, we wonder if we will be able to overcome the challenges it presents. As our loved one's abilities change, so do our challenges. We may have found the solution to one problem and then we are presented with another. It is not always the challenges that present a problem; it is the manner and approach we take in solving them. We must again look at attitude and examine how we are viewing the challenge. If we look at them as defeating, we will be defeated. If we look at them as what they are, only a challenge waiting for an answer, we can triumph over them. Challenges do not have to be an obstacle if we approach them with a winning attitude.

Today I will look at my challenges and see them as a positive initiative ready to be conquered.

Hate

Hate is a powerful emotion, and if we do not handle it properly, it could have destructive results. If expressed, it could lead to depression and anxiety. On the other hand, if it is suppressed the consequence to our loved ones and ourselves could be very destructive. When we are angry, we see only what we want to see and remember only what we want to remember. Hate stops us from thinking, behaving rationally, and seeing situations in true perspective. We need to let go of the past and try to be reasonable. By holding onto hateful feelings, we will only continue to feed them, and they will become more powerful. Hatred serves no purpose, and next to love, it is the most powerful emotion of all. By acknowledging our hate, we can then begin to deal with it in a rational manner and live in the now. Coretta Scott King says, "Hate is too great a burden to bear. It injures the hater more than it injures the hated."

I will not let hate dictate how I feel or what I do. I will acknowledge it and deal with it in a rational manner.

July 4

Influence

As caregivers, we frequently struggle with how to handle the challenging behaviors associated with this disease. Research suggests that caregiver characteristics influence the behaviors of those we care for. If we present ourselves as angry or upset, we can expect our loved one to mirror our outward emotion. If our body language or tone of voice says, we are upset or angry they will react accordingly and become defensive. Our body language represents 55% of our total communication, and it is one of the first things people will react to. It is not always easy to appear calm, but we need to put forth the effort. That being said, we need to understand that most of the time we have a positive influence on them, and we need to give ourselves credit for that.

Recognizing the influence I have over my loved one, I will strive to present myself in a positive manner.

Risks

Taking a risk of any kind can be scary because we are opening ourselves to possible change. We were taught as children to play it safe and not to rock the boat. There are good risks and bad risks. Drinking and driving is a bad risk. As adults, we need to weigh the good and the bad. What is the worse scenario, what is the worst that can happen if I take this risk? Taking risks is not irresponsible as long as we pay attention to the possible outcome, and do not' act on impulse. We need to examine our situation and wait for the real facts before determining whether to take the risk. Going after what we want in life is always a risk but often it is a risk worth taking. Helen Keller was probably right. "Life is either, a daring adventure or nothing at all."

I will not act on impulse and will take risks only after I have evaluated the outcome.

July 6

Music

Music is called the universal language because it connects us with others in a way that words cannot. Music can be a blessing in our time of need. It can sooth us as well as our loved one. It has the power to reduce anxiety and agitation. It can make every day tasks more enjoyable. Music can also provide time for restful healing. Music can be uplifting and can enhance social interaction. It is much easier to perform a task when we are relaxed and feeling well. Our loved one is more apt to follow directions when they are not agitated or fearful. The type of music we listen to is a personal choice. It does not have to be Beethoven or Bach, but our selection should not cause agitation to our loved one. Choosing music we are familiar with will make us comfortable and more receptive to its healing effects.

Today I will reintroduce music into my life and share it with my loved one.

Problem Solvers

Caregivers are great problem solvers, and this disease presents us with many opportunities to use our creative problem solving skills. If they gave a prize for who can solve the most problems in a day, we would take first prize hands down. We may not be able to solve the New York Times crossword puzzle, but we can interpret fragmented sentences and know what they mean. We can adapt every day food to finger food for easier eating. We can tell with a look or a sound when our loved one is in distress and needs our help. We know where to look for creative options and how to overcome obstacles. Our caregiver journey teaches us that no problem is too big or too small if we approach it with an open mind and remain flexible. Approaching our problems with a positive attitude can make our problem solving even more successful.

I take pride in my problem solving skills and will continue to be flexible when searching for a solution.

July 8

Multi-tasking

Multi-tasking means doing more than one thing at a time. It requires that we switch our attention, usually in a rapid manner, from one task to another. Caregivers are the champions of multi-tasking. Typically, it is looked at as a good thing, but as we age it may not be that desirable. One of the problems with multi-tasking is that we become distracted, and could end up feeling out of control. There is no way we can meet our loved one's every need. Studies show that multiple tasking may appear to be more efficient, but it is actually more time consuming, and in some cases poses health risks. Multitasking has its limits. It is OK to stop and regroup before we take on another task. This gives our brain time to recycle and helps us reorganize our thoughts. When we find ourselves trying to do too much at one time, we need to slow down and ask for help.

I will strive to do one thing at a time and do it well.

Change

Change is inevitable in everyone's life. We know that there will be dramatic changes in our loved one as the disease progresses. Even though we know the change is coming, we fear it and sometimes try to ignore it. We rationalize that if we do not think about it, it will not happen. The greatest impediment to any change is the "fear of change" itself. There have been times when we have feared change, only to later have a sense of relief when it happens. Viewing change as always being bad can cause us to feel helpless. When we are receptive to change, we will then see it in a more positive light and be able work through it in a constructive and healthy manner. Preparing for change and not projecting what might be will arm us with the tools to meet it head on and have a more positive result. Change can lead us to new and better experiences if we are open and optimistic.

I will be more open-minded and optimistic about change and not fear or resist it.

July 10

Resilient

Resilient people are able to bounce back after setbacks, failures, and losses. They do not give up and continue to face the future with optimism and courage. Before we can be resilient, we must learn to trust in ourselves. We need to know our strengths and weaknesses. We can never eliminate all the risks or bad things that happen in our lives, but we can learn to deal with them in a constructive manner. Everyone suffers setbacks sometime in their lives. By viewing setbacks as temporary and learning from them, we can move on and take control of our lives. Being resilient does not mean we always have to be strong and should not ask others for support. In fact, being able to reach out to others is what makes us resilient. As the saying goes, when life gets tough the "tough get tougher". When we are resilient caregivers, we have control over our mental well-being and are able to spring back when challenges present themselves.

I will take control over my well-being and be resilient when presented with a challenge.

Spirituality

How we choose to practice our spirituality is a personal choice. We can attend a church service or take a walk in the forest. My grandmother said, "You can pray in a closet and God will hear you." Spirituality takes on many forms. It can be about the spirit or the soul. Expressing spirituality can be beneficial and rewarding for our loved one as well. They have lost so much, and yet most often songs and prayers from childhood will stay firmly rooted in their memory. If we address our spiritual needs and those of our loved one, we will be able to use our faith in coping with the obstacles we encounter. Whether it is the rituals of a church service, the soothing sound of music or the words of a prayer, both we and our loved one will benefit from the expression of our spirituality.

I will use my spirituality to comfort and
sooth my self and my loved one.

July 12

Personal Time

Our personal time is what we make it, but first we must make it. It is easy to say, "I just can't find time for myself." It is sometimes difficult to find the time, but it can be done. There are times when our loved one is engaged in something or is resting. Instead of finding personal time in these moments, we forge ahead with something we think we need to do. STOP! Will the dust still be there ten minutes from now? Of course it will. We need to make our personal time a priority. We need to take this time to do what we want, not what we think we should do. If we do not use this time wisely, it will be gone forever. There is no time like now. We cannot repeat it and we cannot get it back. "Me" time can be the most important time we have for ourselves.

*I will stop making excuses and make
my personal time a priority.*

Lies

We were not raised to lie. Dishonesty and deception were not tolerated in our families. Now we must go into uncharted waters of telling therapeutic lies. We are doing this out of love and empathy for our loved one. We are not doing this out of meanness or because we have done something bad. Our therapeutic falsehoods are loving attempts to help our loved one feel better. We want for them to have the least amount of stress as possible. They have lost the ability to process information and make decisions. We recognize that sometimes a truthful response could be very damaging. Reality orientation will no longer work, and we need to begin using validation. This does not have to be a matter of morality. Does it really matter if they see something as green when it is red?

I will help my loved one in times of need
by validating their feelings.

July 14

Approaches

Our approach in dealing with this disease dictates how well we can cope with it. If we see a problem as cataclysmic, then it will be just that. We sometimes are caught up in the descriptors that are attached to this disease; devastating, tragic, and unending. Yes, this disease is all of these things, but looking at only the negative side of the disease hinders the quality of care we give. If we approach problems as solvable, we will take charge and solve them. This disease forces us to define and refine our approaches in order to have the best outcome and quality of life for us and our loved one. In the end what we are looking for is quality of life, not quantity. The most loving thing we can do for ourselves and our loved one is to approach life as the gift it is.

I will define and refine my approaches that I use in caring for my loved one.

Available Resources

There usually are sufficient resources to fit our needs. The problem is how to access them. By the time we have called five or six numbers and been told by a little polite voice to press 1, 5, or 8, we become so frustrated that we give up. The best action is to go to the source of the most reliable information, the Alzheimer's Association. They are considered the provider of choice when it comes to Alzheimer's and related dementias. They can be accessed by phone or on the web. They have hundreds of brochures on all the pertinent topics. They also have professional, trained counselors to answer our questions and guide us to the appropriate agency or service. We should never be afraid to ask any questions; they have heard it all before. Through proper use of our resources, we can solve many of our problems and find the help we need.

I will look to the resource of choice and
feel free to contact them when in need.

July 16

Personal Hygiene

Personal hygiene seems to be a universal problem when it comes to caring for someone with Alzheimer's. Personal hygiene is something we take for granted. It is something we just do every day without thinking. As our loved one's disease progresses, their ability to do or remember to do basic hygiene becomes diminished and they become more lax in taking care of their personal needs. Unfortunately, we cannot take them at their word, when we ask them such questions as "did you brush your teeth today?" They will probably answer yes, even when they have not. They are not lying because in their mind they did brush their teeth; everyone knows you brush them in the morning. They may even be offended by our asking. We may have to try different strategies before we hit on the one that works in assisting them with their hygiene.

I will approach the topic of hygiene with tenderness and compassion as I assist my loved one in their care.

Guilt

We do not talk about guilt much. It is kind of a personal thing, and if we did talk about it, we would feel guilty about feeling guilty. Guilt does not discriminate. It does not care what color we are, our religion, or our social economic status. A professor or clerk at the seven eleven can equally participate in the guilt trip. Unfortunately, it is almost an inescapable reality for caregivers. So what is this thing we call guilt. It is a self-imposed standard we place upon ourselves. Guilt is a vicious cycle that leads to regrets and self-doubt. No one can make us feel guilty. They may know how to press our buttons but they do not impose the guilt we do. If we are going to work through our guilt, first we have to acknowledge it. Once we recognize guilt for what it is, we can begin to heal and free ourselves of this self-imposed demon.

I will take ownership of my guilt and work on releasing it so that, I can be peace in all that I do.

Regrets

We all have regrets. They are the things we wish we had not said or done, and things we wish we had. We regret we were not able to fulfill some of our dreams. Our minds return again and again to what "might" have been, "could" have been, or "should" have been. We replay the event or image over and over again. By replaying these events and images, we give them fuel to grow. Our regrets hold us back from what we want to do in the present. It is ok to have regrets, as they can be learning tools. It is when we cannot let go of them that they become a problem. We cannot change the past, but we can learn from our past mistakes. If we accept things the way they are and forgive ourselves, we can be freed from the burdens of regret. American Athlete Jackie Joyner-Kersee said it well, "It is better to look ahead and prepare than to look back and regret."

I will forgive myself and move forward without regret.

No

No is such a simple word, only two letters, yet for us as caregivers, it is so hard to say. Sometimes when we do say no, we feel like we have to make an excuse for why we said it. Many times when we say yes to something, when no should have been the answer, we will feel resentment and possible anger at ourselves. The desire to please often prevents us from saying no. The answer no does not have to be aggressive, but it must be firm. We do not have to justify or rationalize why we are saying it. We are only here to serve God, our loved one and ourselves. Trying to do everything can diminish the quality of the time we spend with our loved one. Knowing our limitations will help us in saying no. "No we won't be able to host Christmas this year" is a good beginning. Adding a simple "but we would be glad to stop over at your place for a short time," is a better answer.

I will learn to say no and stop placing myself in situations where I do not want to be.

Defense Mechanism

Denial says I will not believe it, I cannot deal with it, and I do not want to feel guilty about it. Denial can be a defense mechanism that we use to protect ourselves from emotional pain. It becomes a struggle because we are trying to separate ourselves from the situation at hand. When we were children, it was easier to do, but as adults we recognize the consequences of denial and avoidance. The longer we wait, the bigger the problem gets. It seems to take on a life of its own and gathers momentum as time rolls on. These defense mechanisms work for the short run, but not in the long run. Eventually we will have to step up, take ownership, acknowledge it, and deal with it. Then we can commit to a course of action and move forward in our journey.

I will stop using denial as a defense mechanism and commit to a course of positive action.

Ask for What You Need

People are not mind readers. They do not know what help they can give unless we the caregiver let them know what we need. Our needs and desires can range from emotional, physical, and spiritual. We need to remember that we have limits and cannot do everything alone. Forming a support team of family and friends will help lift the daily burdens that lead to stress. If there are no other members of our family or relatives close by, we need to look to friends or members of our church or social group. Finding others to handle family tasks will give us more time to care for our loved one and our selves. Making a list of even the most menial tasks will help us know who is better suited to help in each area. Nothing is too small or big when asking for help. We need to be prepared to be specific when the offer of help is given.

I will look to my friends and family for support and ask for what I need.

Faith

Sometimes when things are not going well, our faith can be shaken. It is difficult to understand why God lets bad things happen. It is ok to waiver in our faith, as long as we get back on track. Our faith will help give us peace and understanding. It will center us so that we can begin our day with love and confidence. It is not our place to question what God's plans are. If we really want to hear God laugh, we might venture to tell him what our plans are! Our fast-food mentality makes waiting even more difficult. As a society, we want instant gratification, and we want it Now. Our timetable is not the same as God's, so we become impatient and think that he does not hear our plea. We need to have faith; he does hear us and will answer when the time is right.

I will stop seeking instant gratification and
have faith that things will happen in good time.

Pride

It is good to take pride in what we do. We are making a difference in our loved one's life. It is when our pride turns into self-rightness that we lose site of our goal. We fail to see our shortcomings and believe that our ideas are better than those of others. We fail to recognize our limitations and push ourselves to exhaustion, both physically and mentally. We are just human and want to do things our way. We may even think ourselves as weak or inadequate if we ask for help. If we fail to recognize our shortcomings, our needs and those of our loved one may go unnoticed. Caregiving is a monumental job and cannot be done just by one person. If we can get past the feeling of self-righteous pride, we can open the door for help. There is a proverb that says, "Pride goeth before a fall." Keeping this in mind, we can put our pride into perspective.

I will not let my pride stop me from asking for help in my times of need.

Feeling Stuck

Most people at one time or another feel stuck in their life. The wheels are spinning, but there is no traction. It may start with a feeling of frustration. We may feel unloved and unappreciated. Whatever the cause, we just do not know what to do at that given moment. We may even fear that we are doing something wrong. When we have these feelings, we also are stuck in repetitive thinking. We continue to have the same negative thoughts and then wonder why things do not change for the better. We need to recognize that these feeling may be a sign that it time for us to make a change. We want to make a change, but our fears over rule us. Instead of becoming overwhelmed when these feelings strike, we need to get back on track. It is not always necessary to take a big leap to move forward. One step at a time can be the best solution.

When I feel stuck in my life, I will draw upon my inner strengths and move on.

Reluctance

We may have taken on our caregiving duties reluctantly. Our lack of enthusiasm may have come out of fear that we were not up to the job, or because our relationship with our loved one was strained and possibly non-existent at that time. This reluctance does not mean we are a bad person. If it comes out of fear of inadequacy, then we can take heart in the fact that there are many resources that can assist us in our newfound role. Strained relationships may be a little more difficult to deal with, but it is far from impossible. Looking back at what caused this distancing; we may be surprised to find that we cannot even remember what caused the problem. We always need to remember that we should never build the wall of resentment and anger so high that we cannot get over it. This may be a good time to heal old wounds.

I will try to heal old wounds and work on
my relationships with my family.

July 26

Collective Voices

Alzheimer's is a disease that seems to always be left behind when it comes to allocating money for research, or the passing of legislature to assist with care. We need to make our collective voices heard. We need to educate legislators about the disease and the devastating effect that will affect our country and its people. Alzheimer's disease needs to come out of the shadows and be seen as the disease of the century. It may be too late for our loved one, but it is not too late for the millions that will be afflicted. We may feel that we are just one person and that our voice is not worth much, but there is power in numbers. If we join our support groups, the Alzheimer's Association and other dementia focused groups, one voice becomes like the "Mouse that Roared." We need to speak up for our loved one because they cannot.

I will join the many voices and advocate for my loved one and all those that are suffering with Alzheimer's.

Activity

It is our responsibility to encourage and initiate activities for our loved one. Their days can be boring if they do not have anything to do but sit or sleep. We need to look for activities that are stimulating, but not too challenging. If possible they should reflect things that our loved one enjoyed in the past. Activities that include their sense of taste, smell, or touch are good to use at any stage of their disease. Most importantly, they must always be "failure free." There is no room for criticism or judgment. One thing to keep in mind is this; TV is not an activity. Too often TV is used as a babysitter. They do not understand what is happening on the TV, and it can lead to further confusion. Alzheimer's affects their motivation so we may have to help them get started in an activity. Well-planned activities can improve the quality of life for our loved one.

I will engage my loved one in activities that are meaningful as well as enjoyable.

Care Dilemma

When our loved one becomes too much for us to care for, we may have to make some difficult choices. There are many alternatives available before we have to choose a nursing home. We can have a person come to our home to assist us. They can also take them out for a walk or ride, which will give us a break, and help stimulate them. Another great alternative is adult day care, a safe place they can go for two or more days a week. Such help will free us up as well as keep them active. There are also assisted livings homes where they can go if they meet the requirements of care. The last is the dread nursing home. We may have heard such bad things that it clouds our judgment. We should never make a decision on hear say. By doing our research and visiting the facilities, we will be able to make the selection with confidence that we are doing the best thing.

I will review all my options when my loved one needs more care than I can give them.

Take a Deep Breath

Breathing…an act that we do approximately 20,000 times a day, can greatly influence our health. There is a connection between deep breathing and stress. Deep breathing provides extra oxygen to our blood and causes the body to release endorphins that can reenergize and relax us. The best part is that we can do it anywhere, at any time, with a little concentrated effort. In eastern cultures it is considered essential to maintaining Chi or life-force energy. In the caregiver world we can embrace this wisdom to help us deal with our caregiver stress. There is no mystery to deep breathing. We do not have to go to the back of the room to a deep corner to do it. By simply sitting or standing straight, inhaling and exhaling slowly and deeply, we can find our Chi, relax, and be more effective in our everyday challenges.

I will learn to use deep breathing in times of stress and maintain my Chi life force.

Social Graces

Our loved one's social graces are beginning to diminish as they progress through their disease. They lose the ability to know right from wrong and at times do things that others see as inappropriate. Their capacity for control is waning. The person we once knew as kind and thoughtful becomes a shadow of their former self. They say and do thing that would be unthinkable if they were their cognitive selves. They say things to others and us that may be hurtful. This can be so disheartening at times that we isolate them so that we can protect them. We do not want to have their feelings hurt. We don't' want others to pass judgment on them. We become embarrassed by their actions and remove them from all social interaction. Protecting them is a noble thing, but we need to let them socialize whenever possible. It is important for them and vital for us.

I will protect my loved one and still let them remain social.

August

❧

"There is nothing that wastes the body like worry, and one who has any faith in God should be ashamed to worry about anything whatsoever"

MAHATMA GANDHI

Advocate

Our loved one can no longer stand up for themselves. They cannot let the people around them know that their disease causes the problems with language or behavior. It is not fair to have people judge them as crazy or mean just because they do not know the situation. It is now up to us to share with others the knowledge we have about the disease. We can help them understand that our loved one is an individual and is not the disease. We need to let people know about our loved one so that they can treat them with dignity and respect. Living with this disease is hard enough without having people make fun or distance themselves because they do not understand the circumstances. When we advocate for them we are showing the devotion and commitment we have for our loved one.

I will advocate for my loved one and share my knowledge of the disease so that others will treat them with respect.

Out of Control

The more out of control we are, the more out of control we get. Sometimes we get ahead of ourselves. Our thoughts jump from one thing to another at lightning speeds. When this happens, we become overwhelmed and step out of the moment. These times do not work well for us. We are so caught up that we try to peak around the corner to see what to expect next. Only we have the power to control how we react in different situations. Slowing down helps give our full attention to what we are doing. By pacing our thoughts, we give ourselves time to make informed decisions and take control of our lives. We all have the desire to live a more balanced, reasonable life, but this can only be done if we slow down. The wise carpenter measures twice and cuts once.

I will make a conscience effort to slow down so that I can enjoy my life now.

Appointments

Having any type of appointment, either for us or our loved one can turn into a challenge. It takes time and energy to get ourselves ready, and even more so to get our loved one ready. When making appointments, we should first try and schedule at a time that is convenient for us. Most often, we do not want to tell our loved one ahead of time, that we have an appointment because it may put undue stress on them. We just want to take them gently when the time comes. There will also be times when nothing works, and we cannot get to the appointment. If we know early enough that we cannot make the appointment, we should call and cancel as soon as possible. However, there will be times when it is out of our control, and making the appointment is impossible. When this happens, we do not have to feel guilty. When it is appropriate, we can call and reschedule.

I will schedule appointments to suit my needs
and that of my loved one.

August 4

Our Support System

When we were young and raising our family, we had a good support systems. We had an inner circle of our family, friends, and neighbors. We took care of each other's children, and were there for them in times of need. Life may have changed, but there are still great sources of support out there. Our family may live far away, but we can still have them in our support system. It is ok to reach out and ask for their help. Our friends may be unfamiliar with caring for someone with memory problems, but that does not mean they would not be sympathetic to our situation. In this day of technology, there are other forms of support as well. There are internet-based support groups, provided by reputable agencies. There are caregiver web sites that address everyday problems. There is a direct care help line manned by professionals of the Alzheimer's Association. It is an 800 number and is open 24/7. We can have the help we need if we just take the time to pursue it.

I will take the time I need to build my support system.

Long Distance Caregiving

Long distance Caregiving can be especially stressful. We want to do what is best for our loved one, and yet we do not feel there is enough time since our visits are very limited. This is why we need to plan ahead so that we can make the best of our time when we do get there. We need to be especially vigilant during this time and observe things such as their personal care, eating patterns, bill paying, and their general safety. We also need to know what support systems are available and how to access them. Being a long distance caregiver is not easy. We need all the help we can get. One of the most efficient types of help is that of a geriatric care manager. They can relieve much of the stress that we feel by acting as a liaison. We need to know what resources are there for us and above all, we must use them.

I will plan for my visit to my loved one so that I can accomplish as much as possible during my time with them.

Celebrate Me

To celebrate one's self is not a selfish act. It is an act of self-recognition that probably is long overdue. Deep in our hearts, we know we are capable of good things. We know that throughout our life, we have made a difference and helped others through difficult times. We have given of ourselves and made a difference in the world. We should never lose sight of who we are or what we have accomplished. As in the past, the things we are now doing are equally important. Our present day caregiving is a powerful statement of who we are and what we can accomplish. We can approach it with confidence and strength. We are not afraid of challenge and welcome whatever mission lies ahead. When we celebrate ourselves, it reminds us of why we are here and keeps us focused on our life's purpose.

Today I will acknowledge the good in me and take a moment to celebrate who I am and all that I am capable of.

Other Diseases

Persons with Alzheimer's are not exempt from other diseases such as cancer and diabetes. Loss of sight or hearing are two of the most common problems merely because of age related change. Loss of sight or hearing can have the most impact on them because it makes it even harder for them to understand and communicate. Distorted perception of sight and hearing makes them more vulnerable to falls and heightened states of confusion. Because they personally do not recognize that they are hard of hearing or have a sight problem, our job becomes a little more challenging. They take their hearing aids out and even throw them away because they do not know what they are. Their glasses are left in some of the strangest places imaginable. It is impossible to monitor them constantly, but we can make sure the hearing aids have fresh batteries and are placed in their ear properly. We can keep their glasses clean, but we cannot keep them from being lost.

I am aware of my loved ones other health problems, and will do all I can to assist them.

Mistakes

Because caregiving is a journey, not a one-day event, we have a lot to do and a lot to learn. As with other areas in our life, we can learn by doing, and by making mistakes along the way. We should not be afraid of making mistakes, its human nature, and we cannot be right all the time. Mistakes are in fact, where the learning is. As the saying goes, "Nothing ventured nothing gained." If we are willing to step out of our comfort zone and try new things, we will learn. It can be a risk, but one worth taking. While making mistakes is a good learning tool, repeating them is not. Success comes from mistakes. George Bernard Shaw agrees and says, "Success does not consist in never making mistakes but in never making the same one a second time." Sometimes we need to make mistakes in order to be ready for the challenge.

I will learn from my mistakes so that I do not repeat them.

Nature

Even nature takes a break in order to replenish and heal. The bears hibernate, the trees defoliate, and they all take a winter siesta. Like the plants in nature, our lives produce best when they rest and are nurtured. There are, however, times when the frost comes early and takes control out of our hands. This is when nature teaches us patience. We learn from nature that we have to be flexible when obstacles present themselves, and if we truly believe in something, we need not be afraid to go out on the proverbial limb. Our roots are strong and we grow through our experiences. We are learning from nature how to move smoothly through life's cycles. We know that in order perform at our best we also need to take time to replenish and rejuvenate. When things get out of control, we have learned to be patience. We may not be the brightest star in the sky, but we do know how to shine.

I will remain strong and remember the
many lessons of nature.

Loving Ourselves

We need to love ourselves all the time, not just when we do something we feel is good. We need to do more than just tolerate ourselves. We can be our own worse critics. Sometimes we treat others better than we treat ourselves. We have more compassion for others than we do for ourselves. We fail to recognize that we are one of a kind, a unique and wonderful human being. We have qualities that may seem invisible to us, but others can recognize them. They may even tell us what a good caregiver and friend we are, but we often fail to hear them, or just brush the comment off. We are all the things others see in us: giving, compassionate, and strong individuals. By practicing self-love and unconditional self-acceptance, we learn to appreciate ourselves and recognize the good that we do for others. The degree to which we love ourselves determines the degree to which we are able to love others.

I will love myself and accept the praises from others.

Overwhelmed

When we are bombarded with too much information or have too much to do, we can become overwhelmed. Now imagine what it must be like for our loved one on a daily bases. Their minds no longer allow them to work through the many steps it takes to complete a task. We think nothing about brushing our teeth we just do it. If we took the time to analyze the steps it takes for this seemingly simple task, we would be overwhelmed. First, we need to understand we need to brush our teeth, and then we would need to find the bathroom. Moving through all the steps, we will find anywhere from 15 to 36 steps that need to perform. Wow, that is scary! Unlike us, our loved one can no longer process what needs to be done or how to do it. If each day seemed new and unfamiliar, we would be fearful and overwhelmed too. By keeping a routine and simplifying the task as much as possible, we can help them become more at ease.

I will find ways to simplify my loved ones everyday tasks.

Touch

Touch is a universal language. Our compassionate touch may be the one thing our loved one with Alzheimer's connects to. The therapeutic value of touch goes back to Greek mythology. Of all the five senses, there is nothing more powerful than touch. By simply holding and stroking our loved one's hand, we show them our love, and give them reassurance that we are there for them. The other benefit of touch can be hydration. Simply applying lotion while we stroke their arms helps to hydrate their skin. The simple act of touch is so versatile that it can be used to relieve stress and calm agitate behaviors. Touch is one of the highest forms of communication that expresses our love and compassion for our loved one. It says, "I love and cherish you."

I will use the sense of touch to communicate my love and respect for my love one.

Hospitalization

When our loved one goes to the hospital, we need to be proactive so that the day of discharge does not come as a surprise to us. Hospital stays are much shorter, and planning needs to start the first day if possible. We need to speak to the doctor and ask about the length of stay. If we cannot get with the doctor then we should contact the discharge planner. Every hospital has a hospital discharge policy. It should include details on how the hospital arranges discharges. The social worker or doctor may not be able to give us the exact timetable, but they can give us an approximate time. We need this time to prepare for special needs that our loved one may have when they come home, or to arrange for our loved one's admission to a nursing home for further therapy. "The best surprise is no surprise."

By being proactive, I prepare for any needs my loved one may have while reducing my own stress.

Tunnel Vision

Many times we get stuck in our line of thinking. We have tunnel vision. We say things like, "I know it will not work if we change it", or "that is the way we have always done it." These are not valid reasons for not trying something new. What is it that stops us from trying new things? Is it that we are afraid to make a mistake? Sometimes we need to do things differently, even if it turns out that we make a mistake and the outcome is not what we had expected. We fight so hard to stay in our comfort zone that we miss the lessons that mistakes can teach us. Even if we do not get it right the first time there's nothing wrong with trying it again. Making even subtle changes in our line of thinking can open a completely new world for us. If we are going to accomplish anything of significance, we need to leave this comfort zone and open ourselves to new and exciting experiences.

*I will broaden my vision and not fear
the changes in my life.*

Life

Why do bad things happen to good people? Why did God let my loved one who is such a good, smart person get dementia? This has been a question that has been pondered by many before us. It seems cruel; life feels so unfair sometimes. If we stop looking at life as being unfair and replace the word unfair with the word adversity it will be easier to find hope and meaning in what we do. If the bad things that happen consume us, we will eventually build up resentment and bitterness towards others and ourselves. If we see ourselves as the victim, our daily life will continue to be a struggle and hinder us from moving on through our adversity. Adversity only has as much power as we give it. Maybe we need to change our outlook on life and move towards the positive. William James was wise in saying, "the greatest discovery of any generation is that a human being can alter his life by altering his attitude."

I will stop being the victim and look at the good things in my life.

Redirect

As our loved one's disease advances, we can expect a decline in reasoning, and judgment. They become more confused and disorientated. These two things alone can decrease their ability to maintain normal behavior. Before we do anything regarding the behavior, we have to ask ourselves, "Is this a problem for me or for them and "is their safety at risk?" Usually the best way to stop the behavior is to redirect them, but before we can do that, we first need to evaluate the situation and search for the cause. Are they in pain, cold, incontinent, or fearful? These are just a few of the questions we need examine if we are going to find the problem. No matter how much we look, we may not find the exact cause. Our best line of defense at these times is to try to redirect them. We can do this by taking their attention off what they are doing and replacing it with something else, that may be pleasurable. It can be a challenge to redirect, but if done in a calm, gentle manner, we will succeed most of the time.

I will be calm and gentle when my
loved one needs redirecting.

Live in the Moment

One mistake we do not want to make is to shortchange the present. If we spend our time worrying about the future and grieving about the past, we will shortchange our loved ones and ourselves. We do not need to forget the past and its lessons. We still should plan, but if we dwell on the past or the future, we will miss the present. The present can be the most rewarding time of all. For the person with Alzheimer's, the most important moment is the present. Their life is only in the here and now. Living in the moment lets us celebrate today. We will be rewarded many times over if we step into their world and live for today. William Penn expresses his thoughts about living in the present: "I expect to pass through this world but once. Any good therefore that I can do, or any kindness or abilities that I can show to any fellow creature, let me do it now. Let me not defer it or neglect it, for I shall not pass this way again."

I will treasure and celebrate the moments
I have with my loved one.

Responsibility

Responsibility is such a strong word, and we take it on as such. Yes, we even take on other people's responsibilities, just so we can get thing done right and on our timetable. We are only responsible for our loved one and ourselves. Because we are a perpetual caregiver, it will be difficult to step back and let others take care of their own responsibilities. People really are capable of solving their own problems, given the opportunity. By trying to solve other people's problems as well as our own, we will surely increase our risk of burnout. Letting people resolve their personal issues can be an act of love. We can save a lot of energy if we stick to our own problems and let others discover their inner strength and find their solutions to their own problems. We need to take care of ourselves first.

*I will take responsibility for myself and
let others care for themselves.*

Documents

We know how important our legal documents are, but it is equally important to make sure the right people have them, or at least know where to locate them. Placing them in a safety deposit box could be a problem. Who has a key and is designated to open it if we cannot? In fact, who knows we even have a safety deposit box and where it is located? All family members that are designated to act in our absence should have all pertinent documents. Any neighbor we trust and are closest to should know where they are in case they need to call 911 for us in the future. Details like these may seem unimportant now but we do not know what the future holds for our loved one or us. Preparedness should always be part of our plan. We need to remember it was not raining when Noah built the ark.

I will alert my family, friends, and neighbors about my legal documents and their location.

August 20

Crisis

Crisis is a good editor. It forces us to stop and think about the outcome. It offers us the opportunity to see the problem and its solution, even if the answer to the problem is not what we want at that moment. If we are delinquent on our light bill, our power will be shut off, and we will be forced to pay the bill if we want light. The journey we are on will have crisis moments, both big and small. Some will be expected and other unexpected. Crisis can mark a real turning point in our lives. These will be the times when we will find out what we are made of. We must not assume that because something is difficult that it is impossible. Caregivers are problem solvers. We have the power to rise above the crisis and make informed decisions.

I will try to avert crisis, but when I cannot,
I will rise above it.

Kiss and Make It Better

When we feel alone and helpless, we want someone to reach out and make us feel better. We want them to kiss our pain and take it away. When we were children, a simple kiss on our "owie" made the pain go away, or at least we thought it did. Of course, it was not the kiss that took away the pain, but rather the comfort and security we felt by being comforted by someone we loved and trusted. This is such a simple gift, one that we can give daily to our loved one. By tenderly kissing them on the cheek or holding their hand, we can help them feel comfort in the moment. Giving our love and affection unconditionally, we can take away the pain, if only for a moment. It may not fix it forever, but for one glorious moment, we have taken away the pain and made them feel secure and loved.

I will show my loved one how much I love them and try to take away any discomfort they may have.

Routines

Caring for our loved one with Alzheimer's, at home is a difficult task, that can become overwhelming at times. Each day brings new challenges as we try to cope with their changing levels of ability. Our loved ones daily routines are very important to them in their deteriorating state. Change is difficult for them no matter what it is. Adults often see daily routines as monotonous and boring, but for persons with Alzheimer's, routines create a sense of security. It helps them know what to expect. Keeping structure helps them maintain their independence longer and makes them feel better about themselves. Their world is turned upside down. Routines are like a security blanket, helping them feel safe and comfortable in their daily tasks. Along with keeping a good routine, we need to remember to be flexible and ready to make necessary adjustment to their routine.

I will create routines in my care so that my
loved one feels safe and secure.

Life's Journey

"All of life is a journey, which paths we take, what we look back on, and what we look forward to is up to us. We determine our destination, what kind of road we will take to get there, and how happy we are when we get there...." Anonymous. Life choices propel us in various directions and define our purpose. Life as a caregiver can be a struggle if we let it. Whoever coined the phrase "Life is a Contact Sport" recognized that if we do not play, we cannot win. The journey of life is just that, a journey. It is not a race or a destination. Instead of wishing away the time, we need to recognize and savor every moment. Our journey may be hard, but the final destination is worth our full participation. We can make it through even the toughest times if we hold onto love and have faith that today can be the best day of our lives.

I will approach my journey through life with love and confidence. I will appreciate every precious moment.

Conflict

We need to work through conflicts together with our families, so that we can better serve our loved one. Although conflicts are common as family members struggle to deal with the situation, they can present a problem when we are trying to get the family together for a family conference. People react differently when faced with the diagnosis of Alzheimer's. Family conflicts can be magnified during this time of stress. We need to keep this in mind and should never let conflict or hidden resentments prevent rational discussion. Ideally, all family members will meet together, and everyone can assume a responsibility. Now more than ever we need to put aside our differences. This could be a very good time to enlist our family's help and heal old wounds. We do not have to agree with our family members, but we need to "agree to disagree," so that we can all move on to caring for our loved one while enjoying our time together.

I will attempt to involve my family in the care of my loved one and work through any conflict we may have.

Nourish Ourselves

We are born people pleaser. We feel the need to put others first. We give so much to others, that we are stingy with ourselves. We sometimes fail to recognize that being selfless with ourselves can eventually turn us into the second victim of this disease. We continue to give until we are drained and exhausted. If we constantly give and do not take time to nurture ourselves, we will eventually burn out. When we deplete our physical and mental reservoir, it leaves us with nothing to give. We must refill our depleted well of energy with compassion and kindness for ourselves. When we care for ourselves, we do not have to feel guilty, nor do we need to justify it. Our health and well-being is critical for the health and happiness of our loved one. We can still be as loving and caring as ever, in fact even more so, because we will have renewed strength to do it.

I will nurture myself, and treat myself with the love and kindness I give to others.

August 26

$Pain$

Persons with dementia do suffer pain, but often they cannot tell us what hurts. Their inability to verbalize how they feel makes it difficult to assess their level of pain. One of the best tools is observation. Our problem solving techniques will again come into play. We need to look at secondary signs of pain such as, increased agitation or irritability, sensitivity to touch, and facial cues such as grimacing. As personal caregivers, we know our loved one better than anyone does. Because of this personal connection, we have the ability to gauge if they are in pain. Pain left untreated could lead to health complications. Pain is nature's way of letting us know our body needs help. Finding the site of the pain and its intensity is pretty much a "hit and miss "situation, but that does not mean we should stop looking. Pain should never be an option for our loved one, and we must continue to investigate and evaluate until we are satisfied that they are comfortable.

Knowing that my loved one cannot always tell me when they are in pain, I will monitor them for any signs of discomfort.

Lingering Regrets

Lingering regrets are usually about things we did not do. Our regrets can pose a problem if we continue to revisit them. When we cannot let go of them, they become a burden. Lingering regrets make us wallow in the past. In the past our youth may have blocked our reasoning. Whenever we give power to regrets, we give them ability to hurt us. We do not have to deny or minimize our actions. We just need to come to terms with them. When our regrets linger, we are stuck in a holding pattern and cannot move forward. We cannot continue to live in the world of "lingering regrets." We cannot turn back the hands of time or erase what we have done, but we can move forward and let go of our past mistakes. If we do not let our pride get in the way, we can trade in the pains of the past for the happiness of the present.

I will not hold on to my regrets. I will move forward and trade in the pains of the past for the happiness of the present.

Wealth

Wealth comes in many forms. To some it is money, to others it is personal possessions, but how valuable are these things if we are not rich in spirit? If we think of wealth as only possessions, we are selling ourselves short. We need to look at the simple things that make us happy today, a smile from our loved one, a phone call from a friend, a song on the radio. Wealth is not complex. It is what we want it to be, simple and fulfilling. Wayne Dyer, author of "<u>The Power of Intention</u>" states "when you change the way you look at things, the things you look at change." Our true wealth comes from the happiness within. The Beatles had it right; "Money can't buy love." By recognizing our personal wealth, we can use it like a bank account and draw upon it whenever we feel down.

I am wealthy many times over, and for that, I give thanks.

Self Care

We do not always pay attention to what our bodies are trying to tell us. We ignore the fatigue and continue to push on. We may need our glasses changed, but who has time for that? If we were to calculate all our self-neglect, we would find that we are the low man on the totem pole. Others needs seem to come first. Like most caregivers, we are perpetual givers. Even though we know this is not good or sensible, we are stuck in the pattern of self-neglect. We were careful to make plans for our loved one so that all of their needs could be met, but what about our needs? Our whole life is not caregiving. We are separate persons from our loved one's illness. We choose to be here because of our love and sense of devotion; we have a duty to care for ourselves.

I will care for myself and pay attention to what my body is trying to tell me.

Wandering

Wandering away from home is among the most unsettling and even terrifying behaviors people with Alzheimer's often exhibit. They are not wandering off to be mean, they simply lack the knowledge to know better. First, we need to see if we can find the reason that initiates the wandering. If we look at their life's pattern we may also find that in their professional life 4 0r 5 o'clock was the time that they left work to come home. Is there too much stimulation in their environment? Are they anxious or distressed? Is there a certain time of day that triggers the wandering? When placed in an unfamiliar setting, they may have a tendency to wander, trying to find where they belong. Whatever the cause is, we need to be prepared. Although about 60% of people with Alzheimer's wander, it is important for all persons with dementia to enroll in Safe Return Program through the Alzheimer's Association before the behavior begins. This programs not only offers peace of mind should they become lost, but it also could save their life.

I will register my loved one in the Safe Return program so that they will be safe and I will have peace of mind.

Clutter

We do not think of those cute little things we got on vacations or gifts from loved ones as clutter. Things are not just things. They usually have an emotional value attached to them. How can we part with them? A good rule of thumb is this: if it has not been used or worn in a year get rid of it. The danger of a cluttered home is that it becomes an obstacle course and unsafe for our loved one and us. We might protest "I am caregiving here; I do not have the time fool around with clutter." By taking just ten minutes, each day to sort and discard unused items we can create an environment that is safer and more peaceful. De-cluttering does not mean just moving things from one place to another. We need to put them away or get rid of them. Being able to find things when we need them is just another bonus. When we de-clutter our homes, we de-clutter our lives.

I will de-clutter my home and make it safe and peaceful.

September

∾

"Courage is not the absence of fear, but rather the judgment that something else is more important than fear."

AMBROSE REDMOON

Anxiety

Anxiety is worry gone wild. When our days are filled with anxiety, it is difficult to accomplish anything or concentrate on things that need to be done. Everyone has anxious moments, but if they are consuming our every thought, they are out of hand. We may dismiss the feeling because we feel that it is o.k. to feel this way. If we do not recognize it, and act on it, we will soon be back in the throes of our old friend Stress, and thus the emotional merry go-round starts all over. When we feel anxious, we need to stop and try to figure out what it is that is causing us to feel this way. Taking care of our emotions is a critical part of our health. We know what problems emotions cause. For the most part, emotional stability will come when we take the time to analyze what is happening and then take whatever steps are necessary to put things back in perspective.

I will stay in touch with my problems and seek solutions
before they turn into anxieties.

It's the Disease

There are times when we think that our loved one is saying or acting out to intentionally annoy us. Even though we know in our hearts that this is not true, it is difficult to rationalize it in the moment. We feel like a target and they are aiming directly for us. We are more vulnerable when we are tired, stressed, or isolated. We take everything personally, and it hurts. It is like living with two other people, one being the person we remember from the past, and the other one that does and says inappropriate things. Knowing that they have lost the ability to reason, we must remember it is not them speaking in an irrational manner. It is the disease. When these moments happen, rather than analyze them, we just need to accept them.

I well strive to remember that the inappropriate things done by my loved one are not personal but part of the disease process.

Taking Life Too Seriously

Sometimes we take ourselves too seriously. We think that we are the only one that can care for our loved one. We do not have time for friends and family. We have forgotten how to enjoy the simple things in life. We cannot remember the last time we had a good laugh. Our life is on a tight schedule, and we do not want to deviate. Small problems throw us out of kilter. Our caregiving journey dominates our life. Personal time for us is non-existent. These are some good clues that we are taking ourselves too seriously. We need to step out of this frame of mind. Having fun or having a good laugh helps us improve the quality of our life. Inner happiness is what propels our sense of creativity. The world does not revolve around us, and that is a good thing. There is nothing so serious in life that it needs to take over and rule how we live. It is time to have fun and let our hair down.

I will strive for inner happiness and stop taking myself so seriously.

September 4

Medication Administration

In the early stages of the disease, it is imperative that we somehow begin to monitor our loved one's medication. Just because they say they took their medicine does not mean they did. They are not lying; they believe that they did, and that we are a ninny for even asking such a dumb question. It is the invasion of their personal independence that causes them to become angry. We need to tread carefully in our attempt to help them with the administration of their medication. It may be helpful to assist them set up a weekly system, keeping in mind that no method is fail-safe. We will need to monitor their self-administration in the beginning of the disease. Later on, we will have to take over the administration entirely, but for now, a gentle reminder should help keep the problem in check.

I will monitor my loved one's administration of their medications and assist them in the most compassionate way possible.

Negativity

Because of our hectic and busy lives as a caregiver, we sometimes lose sight of the things that are positive in our lives. When we worry or become upset over things, we make them appear bigger than they really are. A negative attitude is self-defeating. One of the most important decisions we make in our lives is the attitude we choose to have each day. Attitude comes from within us. Negative thoughts lead to anger, sadness, or depression. One of the worst side effects of a bad attitude is stress. Stress turns into anxiety and then leads to depression. The first step in overcoming negative thinking is to become aware of our thoughts and their effects on us. We can then move on to taking the negative energy and directing it into positive power. Negativity attracts negativity. It is important to practice positive thinking, to recognize that we are valuable people who can achieve remarkable things.

I will overcome my negative thinking and
replace it with a positive attitude.

September 6

Slow Down

In today's world, it is believed that if we move faster, work harder, and do not waste a minute, we will be a success in all we do. We seem to be moving in "fast forward" all the time. Even technology is programmed to help us in this frantic way. We have speed dial, e-mail, text messaging and the list goes on and on. First, we must learn to pace ourselves and stop rushing as though our very life depends on how much we can squeeze into one hour or day. When we work in fast forward, our lives begin to get out of balance. We do not take the time to appreciate the moment. By slowing down, we can develop an awareness of who we are and what we desire. We can learn to reconnect with ourselves and live each day to its fullest. Maybe it is time we heed the song by Simon and Garfunkel recorded in the sixties: "Slow down, you move too fast. Got to make the morning last..."

I will slow down the pace of my life and
stop rushing to get things done.

Depression

As our loved one's abilities decrease, our responsibilities increase. The impact of their disease can prove detrimental to our health. We often sacrifice our own physical and emotional needs, resulting in feelings of anger, sadness, and a high level of stress. These feelings in excess can lead to depression. Depression is not a sign of weakness, rather it is a sign that something is out of balance. Often others will tell us to "just snap out of it", or we may come to believe it is all in our heads. Ignoring or denying our feelings will not make them go away. We first have to look at how we can balance our needs. However, when these feelings become overwhelming too intense, or last for an extensive period it may be time to seek professional help. Depression can be one of the loneliest experiences in our life.

I will not ignore my feelings. I will keep my balance so that I do not fall into a state of depression.

Bad Things Happen to Good People

Why do bad things do happen to good people? This has been a question asked for centuries. When bad things happen to our loved one or us we may become angry with God. Our spiritual foundation is shaken. Given time, we may be able to right the problem, or we may recognize that the problem was not as bad as we thought. Either way, we need to stop asking why something happened, and ask what can we do now that it has happened. We have the freedom to make right or wrong choices, and we will have to deal with the consequences. The Buddha's words paraphrased are: when someone is shot with an arrow, it is better to tend to the wound first rather than asking who shot it. Our belief system should offer us comfort and the best news is that even though we may blame or question God doesn't hold a grudge.

I will stop asking why and begin to ask how can I help now that it has happened.

Over Thinking

In our quest to be the best caregiver ever, we sometimes over think things. In reality, some things are what they are nothing more, nothing less. When we take a problem and over think it, the problem takes on a life of its own. Not everything needs to be dissected. There are times when we get stuck, and we can't stop thinking about a certain problem. This can lead us to excessive worry and a feeling of hopelessness. When we really are caught up in this type of obsessive thinking, we stop trusting our own instincts. Our only solution is to STOP. Stop what we are doing and take action. Over thinking a problem is like beating a dead horse. Maya Angelou sums it up well: "Sometimes things are what they are; Nature has no mercy at all. Nature says, I am going to snow. If you have on a bikini and no snowshoes, that is tough. I am going to snow anyway.

I will stop over thinking my problems and simplify them to meet my needs.

September 10

Joy

There are times when we can really feel the joy in our hearts. We are overflowing with happiness and a sense of well being. We cannot wait to share how we feel with others. We should remember these moments and examine what it was at that time that made us feel that way. Recognizing what makes us happy gives us the opportunity to be more thoughtful in what we do in our daily life. It enhances our ability to feel good and focus on the positive in our lives. When we are joyful, our life flows smoothly. We embrace where we are now, and not where we could be tomorrow. Babies often feel joy because they are always in the now. They do not have the ability to worry about the future. This may be a good time to reconnect with that inner child. Happiness repeated is joy at its best.

*I will look for my moments of joy and
celebrate them to their fullest.*

Decisions

Throughout our lifetime, we will make many decisions, and eventually we may have to make the decision of all decisions, Placement. Chances are that we have made the promise that we would never put our loved one in a nursing home. We meant well at the time and could not envision our life as it is now. For each person the breaking point is different, but the results will be the same. We will feel guilty and angry with ourselves because it has come to this. When we can quietly examine our decision, we will understand that their care simply exceeds our ability and that is OK. It is nothing to feel guilty about. If we have done some preparation ahead of time, it will help. Our loved one can no longer release us from this promise, but we can. We can forgive ourselves and stop feeling guilty. When we do this, we allow ourselves more quality time to spend with our loved one.

I will forgive myself when I have to go back on a promise and know that I have done the best I could.

September 12

Memories

Memories are precious moments from our past. We sometimes are afraid to look back at these memories no matter how good they may be. We feel guilty when we look back at the fun times we used to have together. As our loved one's memory fades, our past memories will be all that we have left. Reminiscing is good, and our past can hold some beautiful memories. We need to hold on to them and embrace them. Memories are a way of holding onto the things that we love and cherish. Our memories also keep us in touch with what we have accomplished in our life. Life will be sweeter if we focus on our good memories, rather than our many challenges. Mitch Album in his book The Five People You Meet in Heaven says, "Memories become your partner. You nurture it. You hold it. You dance with it. Life has to end, Love does not."

I will reflect on my memories and celebrate them
as a testament of my love.

Stress

Stress is the number one problem for caregivers. When caring for a person with dementia, we are prone to suffer higher levels of stress that can lead to serious health problems. If we cannot remember the last time we really felt relaxed, then our stress may be starting to interfere with our physical and mental health. If we feel tired most of the time, if we isolate our loved one and our self, we are showing signs that our stress level is getting out of control. Learning to recognize the signs of stress will help in taking action to reduce our odds of having illnesses that stem from stress. No one can avoid all stress, but we can counteract it by learning how to use some relaxation *techniques.* There is no single relaxation technique that is best for everyone. We need to find the one that best suits our needs. In addition to the calming physical effects of relaxation, it also increases our energy and focus.

I will release my stress by practicing
good relaxation techniques.

Mortality

It is not "if I die", but "when I die." Some people have a hard time with mortality and their eventual passing to the "happy hunting grounds." If we cannot recognize death, then how can we utilize our life to its fullest? For everything there is a beginning and an end, but it's what we do with the middle that counts. If we accept that death is a part of life, there is no need to fear it. Is it the actual death we fear, or is it the fear of the unknown? Because we are perpetual caregivers we always want to be in control, but there are times in life, such as death that are out of our control. Instead of spending time worrying about death, it is best if we learn to treasure life while respecting death. If we come to terms of our mortality, we will be able to lead a more meaningful life.

I will come to terms with my mortality and
treasure life while respecting death.

Self Love

Is loving ourselves first a selfish act? Many of us feel guilty if we put ourselves first, but the truth of the matter is we cannot continue to give to others if we do not give to ourselves first. We all self criticize, and sometimes it seems that our critical voice is louder than our compassionate voice. We set ourselves up for failure if we let our critical voice be the dominant one. The critical inner voice can stomp on our self-esteem and self-image. Only we have control over our inner voice. When we take the time to reprogram our inner voice, we can begin to replace the negative thoughts with positive ones. The result increases our self-esteem and confidence in all that we have and do. By being aware of this critical inner voice, we are taking the first steps in replacing it. By speaking kindly to ourselves, we allow other to see the good in us.

Through my self-love, I will conquer my critical inner voice.

Parents Parent

When we are the child caring for one of our parents, there is a shift in our family roles. The progressiveness of the disease and the constant changes in their needs put them in a vulnerable position. No one wants to be dependent on another person. One of the most important things we must always remember is we cannot be our parent's parent. No matter what, there will be times where we cannot separate ourselves from the child-parent relationship. We will always be daddy's little girl or the favorite son. We want to do all we can to help our parents, but we sometimes find it difficult to cross the invisible line. If we think of it not as a changing role, but more as a change in our function, it may help us to adjust better to the change. We show our children how to care for us by the example we set in caring for our parents.

I will care for my parent as they cared for me.
It is the purest form of love.

Self-Forgiveness

In order to forgive for ourselves, we first must recognize the problem and take ownership of it. It has nothing to do with worthiness. We all are worthy. When we forgive ourselves, it lightens the burdens we carry and helps us move on in our process of self-healing. Self-forgiveness is a choice. If we continue to carry the burdens of our life and berate ourselves, we will not be able to move on in our process of healing. Forgiveness is a very powerful act, which can have wonderful healing effects on our mind and body. Self-forgiveness is the highest form of self-respect. If we accept our humanness, we have taken the first step towards forgiveness. Most importantly, if we cannot forgive ourselves we cannot forgive others.

I will use the act of self-forgiveness to heal me and help me emotionally.

Adjustments

Being a caregiver requires all sorts of mental adjustments. We thought the days of spilled milk were over with the maturing of our children. Now we struggle with multiple demands and problems in caring for an adult. We are juggling responsibilities like never before. We have lost much of our companionship and intimacy that we once shared with our loved one. Even though this all sounds grim, we can rise to the challenge. We care for our loved one out of love and compassion. Change can be difficult, and we will have to make many modifications during our caregiver journey. If we learn to concentrate on our strengths and focus on our accomplishments, we can bring joy to our caregiving. Before we resist change, we should try to think of new angles and modifications that will benefit us both.

I will learn to adjust to change and
"not cry over spilled milk."

*I*ntuition

Intuition is sometimes called the sixth sense. It is also referred to as having a gut feeling. No one ever gave us lessons in caregiving, and sometimes we must trust those gut feelings. Our past relationship with our loved one gives us a sixth sense of sorts. We have a past connection and know their likes and dislikes. Sometimes when faced with a problem, we just know instinctively what we should do. We cannot always put into words what it is we feel. We may not have a concrete reason for these feelings, but they are strong enough that we feel comfortable to act on them. It can also be a matter of faith and trust in our higher power and in ourselves. When we begin to trust our inner feelings, we will be able to rationalize these intuitive thoughts, thus making better decisions. Our intuition is a source of guidance that, if nurtured, can lead us in the right direction.

I will honor my intuition and let it
guide me to better decisions.

September 20

Stages

There are many ways of looking at the stages of the disease Alzheimer's. Some people believe there are seven stages of the disease while others believe there are just three. It really is a matter of opinion. The problem with trying to stage a person is that this is not a "one size fits all" disease. Not everyone will experience the same symptoms or progress at the same rate. We try so hard to understand what is going on. We do research to find out just what is going to happen in the future. The problem with this is we tend to project. If we find out that they could have a certain behavior in the future we project and worry unnecessarily. The key words are could have. Maybe they will have that behavior, and maybe they will not. It will be easier if we just take one day at a time. There is enough to think about without trying to project the future.

I will stop projecting and take one day at a
time enjoying them as they come.

Journaling

Journaling is a good way to put our thoughts on paper. It is a diary of sorts. Writing down our inner most thoughts helps us to clarify them. The mere act of putting thoughts into writing is in itself a stress reliever. We can gain self-knowledge about ourselves. We can also work with our thoughts in new and creative ways. It is said that journaling stimulates creativity. It gives us the opportunity to look objectively at what is happening in our life. Then we can use it for self-direction. A problem written on paper may not seem as bad as our minds have led us to believe. We do not need to write a book; a few sentences about how we feel about a stressful event may be enough to guide us back to more rational thinking and problem solving. The smallest moments can become precious when preserved in our journals.

*I will use my journaling skills to help relieve my stress
and record my important thoughts.*

September 22

Opportunity

When opportunity knocks, do we answer? When a friend or family asks, "what can I do?" do we tell them? When we know our available resources, do we use them? When we feel sick, do we make a doctor's appointment. Do we look to our church, which was always a place of comfort for us, for assistance? We have many opportunities, but we do not always take advantage of them. We may fear that by asking for help we will appear weak. Our fear of being rejected could also be holding us back. Whatever the reason, it is not valid enough to stop taking advantage of the opportunities that are available to us. Not taking advantage of opportunities is opportunities lost. <u>In Life's Little Instruction Book</u> H. Jackson Brown, Jr. tells his son "nothing is more expensive than a missed opportunity."

I will look at the opportunities that can assist me and use them to the best of my ability.

Cake

Who said we could not have our cake and eat it too? We are the sandwich generation. We are mothers, spouses, friends, and sometimes even the breadwinners. Can we fulfill all these roles? Yes, if we learn how to ask for help, how to say no, and most importantly, how to be good to ourselves. We do not have to make a sacrifice of something we like to do or choose between the greater of two evils. It is all about quality not quantity, and it is a delicate balancing act. We know who we are and what we are capable of. If we look at the division of our lives and the balance we need to maintain, we can be successful, as long as we do not cross that invisible line and try to be all thing to all people. The question remains, "what good is cake if you cannot eat it?"

I will stop trying to be all things to all people,
and seek balance in my life.

September 24

Pleasure

Caregiving does not always have to be about bathing, dressing, eating, and other daily tasks. It is a good idea to do things that will bring pleasure to our lives and theirs. Life often seems short, because we are trying to rush through it and do not take the time for simple pleasures. It is like the old cliché's "take time to smell the roses." Keeping pleasure in our daily lives helps to stave off stress and depression. Pleasures can range from the simplicity of drinking a cup of flavored cappuccino to taking a walk through the mall, and of course, we cannot forget the simple pleasures of nature. When we feel pleasure, our loved on can sense it, and they will react to our positive state of mind. Being a caregiver does not mean we have to give up life's pleasures; we just need to plan for them better. Psychologist Joseph Campbell is widely known for his favorite rule for living: "Getting your bliss starts with finding the bliss where you are."

I will slow down and seek the pleasures in my everyday life.

Getting a Good Nights Sleep

When our nights become quiet, our minds begin to take us on a journey through our world of what needs to be done, or what we should do. Why is it that our mind is more active during this time? The fact is, it is not; it just seems like it is because when we are relaxed, we are more aware of it. For some reason our mind tends to go into the problem solving mode at the end of the day. We have the ability to redirect these thoughts, but it will take some refocusing. Using soft music, a miniature fountain, or even the ticking of a clock may be just enough sound to re-focus us. Staying up to 3 am, worrying about our problems will only make sleep more difficult. It is important that we get a good night's sleep. Sleep is essential for our health and well-being.

When my mind goes into over drive at night, I will refocus so that I can have good nights sleep.

Positive Emotions

We control our emotions. Our state of mind takes its lead from how we react to our emotions. It is impossible to be in a positive state of mind all the time, but if we are in a bad mood, nothing will seem right. Our problems seem bigger, and we lose perspective of the whole picture. Changing how we feel is done in baby steps and with great thought. By changing our negative thoughts into positive ones, we take the first step towards contentment. All too often, we look for what is wrong or obsess about our imperfections, and we refuse to acknowledge the good person we are. Positive emotions will help us affirm the goodness in ourselves. We will be the person we want to be and the person that others want to be with. The world is imperfect, and we are imperfect, but that should not stop us from thinking positively.

I will affirm my positive thoughts and
move towards contentment.

Arguing

Arguing with a person who has Alzheimer's will not only be unproductive but also ineffective. This disease not only robs them of their memory, but also of their ability to reason. We may think that they are being obstinate on purpose, when actually they are afraid and fearful about what is happening to them. Above all, we need to always remember that just because they have dementia does not mean they do not have feelings. No matter what stage of the disease they are in, they can sense tension and conflict. We need to avoid conflict at all costs. Arguing and confrontation can cause them to be agitated and defensive. We probably did not win the arguments before they had this disease, but we really will not win now. Take the path of least resistance or just do not say anything. Agree with them while offering the reassurance that everything is ok.

I will avoid arguing and confrontations with my loved one.
I will use reassurance and validation to comfort them.

Wholeness

Wholeness is a state of mind where we feel content and fulfilled with who we are, and what we do. It is believing in ourselves. Sometimes it is difficult to recognize our wholeness because our lives are often fragmented. By looking at what works in our life, and what does not, we can begin to focus less on what is missing in our lives and recognize what we still have. When we feel whole, we can better deal with the difficulties of life. By taking control of our lives, we begin to recreate the person we are. We will feel content and have a sense of well being. When we nourish our body and soul, we make ourselves whole and complete. Feeling complete is a step toward full happiness. As Dr Phil says, "I want you get excited about your life."

I will believe in myself and get excited about my life.

Burnout

Caregiver burnout is a state of physical, emotional, and mental exhaustion that can be accompanied by a change in attitude. Others may see the signs of our burnout before we do. Caregiver burnout does not just happen. The total sum of all the work and responsibilities, along with physical and emotional exhaustion, equals burnout. All caregivers will suffer some degree and form of burnout, but what we do not want to happen is to, crash and burn. We are the only ones that can take control over these times. First we need to recognize the signs. The signs may not seem like much individually, but together they are the right formula for disaster. Sleepless nights, outbursts of anger, isolation, and emotional or physical exhaustion are all contributing factors. In order to avoid burnout, we need to use every resource available to us to get our life back in balance. If we are observant, we can be forewarned and hopefully avoid the pitfalls of burnout.

I will be watchful for the signs of burnout
and heed its warnings.

October

∽

"Thousands of candles can be lit from a single candle, and the life of the candle will not be shortened. Happiness never decreases by being shared."

BUDDHA QUOTE

Balancing Act

The responsibility of our everyday caregiving duties, along with taking care of our self, doing our household chores and all the things we need to do to survive is a delicate balancing act. It is not the act of balancing that is important, but how we perceive the responsibilities. We need to take each day as it comes, knowing that we cannot be all thing to all people. We have a tendency to try to do it all. One of the most helpful things we can do to keep things in balance is to delegate. There are people that want to help. We also need to recognize that it is ok if we do not accomplish all we had set out to do each day. There are times when we need to choose one task over another. If we have confidence in our abilities and are willing to accept change, we will be able to approach this balancing act with strength and confidence.

If I do not accomplish all that I set out to do today, it is OK. There is always tomorrow.

Chaos

In the middle of chaos, it is hard to find peace. Life as a caregiver is a challenge. When the phone will not stop ringing or we feel like there are not enough hours in a day, chaos begins to reign. Usually the chaos is of our own making. We take on more than we can handle. We do not ask for help. We sometimes blame others because it is easier to shift the blame. Chaos also presents itself when we have conflicting priorities. We have so many things on our "to do list" that we cannot decide what to do first. By taking ownership of the things we will be able to move beyond the physical and emotional chaos that is plaguing our life. Problems will be solved and things will begin to make sense. To make sense out of chaos, we must own it before we can regain control.

*I will take ownership of my problems and
begin to solve them.*

Creativity

When we were very little we were taught to color inside the lines. This was one of the first lessons in following directions. However, in the beginning we did not stay in the lines, not because we did not want to, but it was hard since we did not have the hand-eye coordination. Who is to say that staying with in the lines is good or bad, right or wrong? Caregiving is hard, and there are many times when we must be creative and go outside the lines. If our loved one has a problem with bathing, we need to get creative and turn it into a spa experience by making the room warm and inviting, and introducing some aromatic fragrance. It is all creativity. In the caregiver world it is called "doing whatever it takes." By being creative caregivers, we can make and solve most problems with solutions that work for both of us. We must also keep in mind that what worked today may not work tomorrow.

*I will use my creativity to help find solutions
to my everyday problems.*

Plan

When we hear the diagnosis of Alzheimer's or dementia, it sends our golden years planning into a tailspin. We now need to make different plans for the future, and one of the most important is end of life issues. If our loved one is in the early stages, they may be able to express their wishes, but this of course, is not always the case. However, we must remember to be empathic, caring, and realistic when approaching these issues. Our loved one's needs will be ever changing, and if we have done advance planning will we be more capable of giving them the support and comfort that they need. Planning will also give us the opportunity to avoid going into the crisis mode when our loved one's condition or needs change. Fortunately, we do not have to do these things alone. There is much information on the internet and through the office on aging that can help guide us through.

I will set a plan for my loved one's care, and take pay attention to all the details.

Projecting

We need to live in the now because we cannot predict the future. In reading, self-help books, we try to find our circumstance and look for help in solving a problem. Looking for what will happen next to our loved one as they progress in their disease may not be as helpful as we think. No two people present the same in a disease process. If we have seen one Alzheimer's patient we have only seen one Alzheimer's patient. For example wandering is a common problem in Alzheimer's patients, but the truth is not all will wander. To project into the future about things that may happen to us or our loved one consumes too much energy and sets us up for failure. We are wiser to address current problems and try to solve them before we move onto tomorrow's perceive problems. We need to work with the problem of today and let tomorrow be tomorrow.

I will try not to project the future and live
for the blessings of today.

Doctors Appointments

When we have a doctor's appointment we often leave without getting our questions answered or understanding what the doctor has told us. Since doctors have a limited time to spend with us, we should prepare for the visit by doing some of the following: Make lists of all medications taken, including over the counter medications. If the appointment is for our loved one, the doctor should be informed that we have a durable power of attorney for their healthcare so that they will speak directly to us. If we do not understand what the doctor is saying, we need the doctor to explain it to us until we do. Keeping a journal of our loved ones behavior will help the doctor understand where they are in their disease process. If our loved one becomes agitated later in the day, also known as Sundowning, we should schedule the appointment for later in the day so the doctor can observe the sundowning problems they are having.

I will prepare for each doctor's appointment so that all my questions and concerns will be answered to my satisfaction.

Respite

Respite can be looked at as an adult time out. We face many challenges in our 24-7 journey. We need relief, be it a day or two or an extended time away from our loved one. If we do not do this, we may be heading for trouble down the road. Respite can be a time to refuel our energy or just kick back and relax. Whatever type of respite we choose, we need to recognize, it is only partially for us. Our loved one will also benefit when we have renewed energy and faith. One of the benefits of respite is decreasing our old friend stress. We need to take this time with out guilt. If we succumb to guilt, we are negating the purpose of our deserved time out. Using our resources and planning our respite time well can be the best gift we can give to our loved one and ourselves.

*I will plan for respite time for myself so that
I can refuel and reenergize.*

October 8

Humor

It is not that humor is not around us during our caregiver journey; it is that we will not let it in. Laughing and crying provides an outlet for stress. Humor is a coping mechanism. If we take things too seriously and fail to see the humor, we will propel ourselves into an emotional state that could lead to depression. If we learn to laugh at ourselves and not take everything seriously, we will be happier and more relaxed. When we recognize the humor in a situation and laugh, we are laughing at the situation and not at our loved one. We need to be cautious as to when and how we laugh, so that our loved one does not feel that we are laughing at them. Funny things do happen in life and there will be moments where we can laugh with them. Humor is good for the body and great for the soul.

Today I will try not to take everything too seriously, and I will find a reason to laugh.

Stealing

Having our loved one accuse us of stealing from them is a common problem faced by many caregivers. It is bad enough that we put things away ourselves and then cannot remember where we put them, but to be accused of hiding or stealing things puts the frosting on the cake. The fact is they have put them somewhere. A person with memory impairment is not necessarily hiding things. They just want items to be safe. If we are accused of stealing something, we should not take it personally. Arguing with them or mentioning their memory problems is cruel and serves no purpose, and attempting to deny the accusations may only make things worse. If they accuse us of taking something, it is best to offer our assistance in finding it. If their agitation continues, we should remove ourselves from the area or take the blame and move on.

I will attempt to find my loved one's favorite
hiding places so I can help them find things when they
believe they were taken or lost.

October 10

My Mother

Are you my mother? This is a very cute and sweet question when asked by the little bird in the Dr Seuss book "<u>Are You My Mother</u>." That question asked now by our loved one can be heart breaking. Forgetting people or things is common for people with this disease, and it is especially difficult when the forgotten person is us. They have not really forgotten us. What is gone is their visual perception of exactly who we are in the structure of their life. When this happens, it can rock our world. Even though we expect these types of questions as the disease progresses, we are never really prepared for them. It is how we answer these questions that counts. Setting reality aside and validating them will work the best. Take a deep breath. "Yes I am your mother and I love you very much."

I will be gentle in answering the questions my loved one has, especially if it involves our relationship together.

Emotional Exhaustion

There are times when we cannot even think straight, and the mere thought of performing even the simplest task is overwhelming. It may not be a physical type of tired, but a mental one. Everything seems out of order and we cannot wrap our thought process around where to begin. These are times when our inner self is screaming, "Slow down, ask for help, and take time out." Even at these dire times we do not always listen, and later we wonder why things are falling apart around us. Unfortunately, our days will continue to be a struggle if we continue to ignore these inner warnings, but if we heed them, we can save ourselves a lot of grief. When we are suffering emotional exhaustion, we need to refuel our bodies and minds and do whatever it takes to get ourselves back on track. Listening to our inner self can be considered a tool for wellness and help us keep our life in balance.

I will do whatever it takes to keep myself from being emotionally exhausted.

October 12

Kiss Principle

The "Kiss Principle" is an acronym for "keep it simple stupid," and this can be applied to our daily lives. To achieve our goals we often move too fast. We do not stop to think things through, thus we add unnecessary pressure and make things more complicated than they need to be. Confucius says, "Life is really simple, but we insist on making it complicated." The more complex our lives become, the more we crave simplicity. Making our daily life simple is not always that simple. We have many things in life that distract us, but when we know our priorities, we can make the process of finding simplicity much more attainable. By taking the extra time to think a project through, we will not only maximize our time but also simplify our lives. We need to stop worrying about things that are out of our control and stop making thing so complicated. If we simplify our lives, just a little, we eliminate some of our stress.

I will work at simplifying my life and take
it one-step at a time.

The Future

As we age, the future is now. We have more years behind us than we do ahead of us. If we look only to the past, we cannot live in the present. We may have taken on this position of caregiving reluctantly. The relationship with the one we are caring for may not have always been pleasant. They may have been verbally or physically abusive to us. What ever the past problem was, we now face a moral dilemma. What ever is past is gone and cannot be changed, and when we dwell on it, we set up roadblocks that will interfere with the present. Our loved one has lost the ability to reason so having a therapeutic conversation with them is not possible. This problem may never be solved, so we need to decide if we are up to caring for them. If we answer yes, then we have to put the past to rest and start anew.

I will forgive the past and live only in the future so that I can give the best care possible.

October 14

Behavior

We know that at times our loved one acts in a childish manner. We even label their behavior as bad or unacceptable. However, before we label their behavior in a negative way, we must first examine it and determine if it is really bad. Are they going to harm themselves or others by acting out, or is it just inconvenient or unacceptable for us? When inappropriate behavior is exhibited in public, it can be embarrassing. It will take all we have to stay calm and not get angry. Our best defense is to attempt to refocus or redirect them. When this does not work, it may be best to remove them from the situation. Foremost, we need to remember that they do not understand that what they are doing is wrong. This truly is a time where we need to pick and choose our battles.

Today I will step back, look at my loved one's behavior, and determine if it is my problem or theirs.

Asking Why

In the past asking our children "why did you do that" was a futile question because we knew the answer would be, "I don't know." Asking our loved one questions, Who, What, Where or Why is also futile. Our loved one is losing the ability to think logically, so they do not have the ability to answer the "W" questions. By asking these questions in an attempt to communicate, we can make them feel more confused and fearful, especially early on in the disease when they recognize that something is wrong but do not know what it is. Why is an open-ended question and requires memory and logical thinking in order to answer. These "W" words are best left to newspaper articles or invitations. Most of the time it just does not matter; again, it is what it is. We do not want to make them any more fearful in their already confused world.

I will eliminate who, what, where, and why from my speech when communicating with my loved one.

October 16

Singing the Blues

Most people like to hear the Blues sung at a jazz festival, but to hear it during a private conversation can be very annoying. If all the bad things that are happening dominate, our conversation our audience will soon be limited. This is not to say that we cannot talk about our problems sometimes, but we need to choose the time carefully. Whining is not a pleasant thing to listen to, and done on a regular bases can cause our family and friends to avoid us; then we will truly become isolated. When someone unloads his or her problems on us, we do feel uncomfortable. Singing the Blues or complaining is counterproductive. It has been said that, 90 percent of the people do not care about our problems ... and the other 10 percent are glad it is us instead of them. There is a difference between singing the blues and talking constructively about our caregiver lives.

I will try not to complain and will use
my conversation constructively.

Mixed Emotions

There are times when we play emotional ping-pong with ourselves. We go from angry to happy to hurt, all in a short period. Family members and friends do not understand these fluctuating emotions and may begin to criticize us for being too emotional. We need to remember that they are not in the trenches of caregiving twenty-four, seven. They will never understand until they have walked our walk. The saying goes, "the person furthest away has the most to say." Their criticism can lead to even more wavering emotions. This may be a good time to enlist their help. We should invite them to stay with our loved one for a couple of days while we go away for some much need rest. If this ploy works, it will give them the opportunity to see first hand what our caregiver life is like, and understand why we are sometimes tired and irritable. This may also inspire them to offer some help.

I will keep my emotions on a level keel and use my creativity to solve my problems.

Time

In caring for someone with memory impairment, we soon find out that time, as we know it, does not have much meaning for them. Days bump into nights, causing them to be confused and agitated. They do not sleep well at night, and when they sleep during the day, we feel guilty if we do not use that time productively to get things done. If they are up three or four times a night, we have to stand vigil to ensure their safety, thus leaving us sleep deprived. If we are sleep deprived, we will not have the patience and energy needed to take care for them. Sleep is an important factor for our health. We need to place more importance on getting the sleep we need so that we can stay well and not fall into the trap of sleep deprivation and its consequences.

I will take time to rest so that I will
not become sleep deprived.

Word Finding

When our loved one has difficulty finding the right word to express themselves, they become upset. How hard it must be to know what you want to say, but cannot find the word to express it! The gradual loss of communication is one of the most difficult things for us to accept. Substituting a word which is linked by meaning (e.g. Time instead of clock) is common, or they may use a wrong word, that sounds similar (e.g. boat instead of coat). Even though they have problems speaking or understanding the spoken or written language, they often retain the rote ability to sing familiar songs. Although there are many facets to this disease, the word-finding problem may be one of the most distressing. If we stay calm and try to understand the message, we may hear a word or two that can help us decipher what they are saying. We are better able to understand if we use our skills as compassionate communicator.

I will use my skill of compassionate communication to communicate better with my loved one.

October 20

The Past

Hemingway said, "You cannot return to your boyhood, because the boy isn't there any more," but for people with Alzheimer's maybe he is. As their disease advances, they begin to revert further and further into the world of their childhood. Our common sense tells us that most people do not live in the past. For persons with dementias this regression is not only normal, it can at times be comforting. Putting aside our common sense, we can step into their world. If they think they are with their mother and feel safe and happy, who are we to try to bring them back to reality? Being sensitive to their world and validating them is a positive approach that can give comfort. When someone we love dies, we may wish we could see him or her for one more day, or even one more hour. Maybe this is a gift from God to our loved one.

When my loved one lives in the past, I will validate and respect where they are now.

Control

We have a difficult time controlling what is happening in our lives now that our loved one has been diagnosed with Alzheimer's disease. We watch them lose control over their mind and body. We become impatient and frustrated. We have a difficult time dealing with our emotions and personal well-being. We feel like our lives are becoming unraveled. As much as we want to be in charge of all that is happening around us, we need to realize that we do not always have to be in control. We waste valuable time over things that are out of our control. It is futile to try to be in control of things that we do not and cannot have control over. We need to admit to ourselves that we can only do so much, and after that, it is up to our Higher Power to take over. When we use our thoughts to control our emotions, we can begin to let go and our burdens will be lightened.

Today I will take control over my emotions. I will let go of things out of my control and put my trust in a Higher Power.

October 22

Night Thoughts

The lights go out; our head lies softly on our pillow, and our eyes close in anticipation of a good night's sleep. Bam! Our brains switch on bombarding us with thoughts of what we did today and what we need to do tomorrow. It's like sitting in a room with 20 people and having them all talk at once. Even though we know we cannot do anything about it at that time of night, it continues to plague us night after night. The problem with this type of thinking is that we play it over and over again without a solution. Albert Einstein said, "Insanity is doing the same thing over and over again and expecting different results." We can attempt to quiet our thoughts, but there is no one solution for everyone; the best we can do is try different techniques until we find one that works for us.

I will use quiet thoughts or meditation to
silence my night thoughts.

Ego

The noun ego is often defined as false pride. There are many times when our egos get in the way. By being egotistical, we only get short-term satisfaction. We become self absorbed in our thoughts and needs. We begin to close our hearts and minds. We shut out those that could help us. Egotism is self-limiting and has a price. Many times, we cannot see or hear what others have to say because we are so engrossed in our own little world. Our untamed egos can get in our way and stop us from having a personal connection with others. "If you want to reach a state of bliss, then go beyond your ego and the internal dialogue. Make a decision to relinquish the need to control, the need to be approved, and the need to judge"…Deepak Chopra By becoming conscious of our egos, we can move away from self-centeredness. If we can let go and let God, even some of the time, our heart and mind will be open to receive the help and love of others.

I will let go of my ego so that my heart
and mind will be free.

Keeping Score

For the most part when we argue with someone, we think it is all about winning. We sometimes even keep score. We want to be right, which means the other person is wrong. This is truly a "no win" situation. It often results in disharmony in the family because feelings are hurt, and someone comes out wounded. Instead of focusing on winning, we need to keep our eye on the goal, of perhaps solving the problem or raising the other person's awareness to the problem. Everything we say and do in these situations should start and end with what is best for our loved one. We are not in a competition. Caregiving is hard enough without making it a competition. The best way to "win" an argument is to aim for a goal other than being right. Sometimes when we win the argument, we can lose the game.

When an argument presents itself, I will attempt to disarm it and keep my focus on the goal of giving the best care possible to my loved one.

Hydration

The importance of staying hydrated can never be over stated. As we age, we do not have the same thirst sensation as we did in younger years. Many times our loved one can no longer recognize the sensation at all, and may even refuse to drink. Dehydration has many effects on the body. It can contribute to bladder infection, constipation, and even increased disorientation. Drinking eight glasses of water, a day is unrealistic for them. The best approach can be to encourage small sips through out the day. There are also many drinks on the market that may please their pallet and help their intake. We can also dip into our bag of creativity and make some delicious blended drinks. By putting a little bit of variety in their life and making the drinking experience pleasurable, we can help stave off dehydration.

I will do whatever it takes to keep my loved one hydrated.

Knowledge

Knowledge is power! Without it, we cannot plan or learn the skills we need in order to care for our loved one. We can flounder with self-doubt and wonder if we are doing the right thing, or we can look for sources that will enlighten us. Knowledge empowers us to take action. There are many good books on the market but <u>The 36 Hour Day</u> by Doctor Rabin is pretty much considered the bible of Alzheimer's self-help books. The Alzheimer's Association also has a wealth of knowledge. They have trained people to talk to on their help line. Their programs and literature are outstanding. The internet also has good information, but we need to be guarded in this arena and know the qualifications of the author. Using these sources as a guide, and not expecting any source to provide the whole answer, will help us in our caregiver journey. The knowledge we gain today may be invaluable tomorrow.

I will seek the knowledge that is available for me and use it to guide me.

It Doesn't Matter

The mask of the statements, "it doesn't matter, or I don't care what other people think" can keep us from exploring our true feelings. The fact is we really do care; we care passionately about what others think or say about us. Using this train of thought is a defense mechanism that can prove to be unhealthy. We cannot hide from our real thoughts. We are not kidding anyone, especially ourselves, when we say these things. We cannot please everyone all the time; we are only human, and we do make mistakes. By recognizing our humanness, we can be more comfortable with what we do and the decisions we make. Everyone wants to be accepted and recognized for what they do, and we should not use this defense mechanism to avoid facing issues.

I will learn to express my feelings in a more positive manner and stop hiding my true feelings.

Mornings

How we start our mornings usually sets the pace and mood for the day. If possible, we should lie in bed for just a few moments and set the foundation for our day. We can use prayer, positive affirmations, or simple visualizing. The short time we take to ourselves in the morning could be, the most positive and productive part of our day because we are laying the foundation upon which we build our entire day. Starting our day in this positive way will take practice since we are used to jumping out of bed and putting our day on autopilot. In preparing for our day, we should not use this special time to problem solve. These moments are best used to quiet our minds and revive our spirits. Today will never happen again if we set the groundwork in the morning; we can enjoy each moment and make them count.

I will lay the foundation of my day by
thinking positively each morning.

Resilience

Being a caregiver for someone with Alzheimer's puts us in a precarious situation. The rules for our personal survival are ever changing. We need to be concerned with the ongoing and ever changing needs of our loved one. We can emerge from our challenges exhausted and bitter or strengthened and enhanced. It is our choice which one to choose, either way our lives will never be the same. Our inner nature makes us strong. Instead of complaining, we embrace the challenge and work through it. We maintain our resilience by coping and adapting to change. We are nonjudgmental and try to stay emotionally flexible. We use every creative outlet we can draw on. Being resilient in the face of adversity, we take responsibility for our actions. Resilience is our positive action that we use to cope with stress. The saying "when things get tough the tough get tougher" appropriately describes us as caregivers.

I will take positive action. I will work through my problems and embrace the challenges.

Uniqueness

We are all unique unto ourselves. No two people have the same DNA. This uniqueness is what makes us individually exclusive. Therefore, to think that all persons with Alzheimer's behave and progress the same would be a contradiction to our individuality. It is important to remember that a person with dementia is still a unique and valuable human being, despite their illness. Although some symptoms of dementia are common to everyone, dementia affects each person differently. People with dementia lose their abilities at different rates. The changes occur in their brain at different rates. In an effort to become a more informed caregiver, we have read many books and do a great deal of searching on the internet. Importantly we must remember that this is not a "one fits all" disease. Our loved one is a unique individual. We need to do everything we can to help them retain their sense of identity and feelings of self-worth.

I will cherish my loved one as the unique
individual that they are.

Therapeutic Fibs

"I've never lied to him in all these years, and I'm not going to start now." This is probably not true but, what ever. It's not about us anyways. Because our loved one lives deeper and deeper in the past they may ask "where is my mother?" "Your ninety years old, and your mothers been dead for twenty years." What a cruel thing to say. Usually these answers come quickly with out thinking; because we cannot even imagine them, believing their mother is still alive. However, to them she is, and by not validate their state of mind we can start a grieving pattern. This is new, news to them. We would be better off to say; "she is not here right now, but I'll call you when she comes" Telling therapeutic fibs, or little white lies, is not an issue of morality when dealing with persons with Alzheimer's. It is simply a form of compassionate communicating used to help decreases their distress.

I will not view therapeutic fibs as a moral issue,
but rather as a form of communication that can make
my loved one feel more comfortable.

November

∽

As we express our gratitude, we must never forget that the highest appreciation is not to utter words, but to live by them.

JOHN FITZGERALD KENNEDY

Dignity

We would all like to age with dignity. Dignity is every person's basic human right. Unfortunately, the word "dignity" has lost its meaning when it comes to caring for someone with dementia. As their disease progresses they will need more personal body care, and that can be the real beginning of their lose of dignity. How would we like it if someone had to shower or dress us? Our bodies are personal and the mere thought of strangers or family seeing us naked, sends a chill down our spine. Therefore, it is true for the most part that, we really do not know what dignity is, until we have lost it. One of the hardest tasks of love for us as caregiver is trying to help them maintain their dignity. Our loved one can no longer fight for their dignity, so it is our duty to see that all care and communication be delivered with the respect that they deserve.

I will be mindful and observant of how people view
and treat my loved one, and demand that it be
done in a dignified manner.

Caregiver Needs

There is something written called the caregiver bill of rights. In short it says I have the right to; Take care of myself, seek help whenever necessary, to express my feelings, to not feel guilty and to make a life for myself. What this is telling us is, we have the right and duty to care for ourselves. We are individuals and we have needs that have to be met. We are the only ones that can make sure our needs are met. With all the unique jobs we as caregivers have to do, and the fact that there never seem to be enough time to do them all, it is sometimes necessary to take a step back and reassess our needs. We are back to the metaphor for taking care of ourselves "take your oxygen first." In other words if we do not take care of ourselves first we will not be able to care for the one we loved.

I will care for myself first, so that I will be there to care for my loved one.

Ready or Not

Ready or not, here I come, this is a verse we know well from our childhood. In the world of caregiving, it can apply to how prepared we are, for an illness of our own. If we become ill, and we will at sometime, who will take care of our loved one. It could be for a day or a week, either way we need to have a plan. We tend to think of ourselves as infallible, like we did as a teenager. We can handle anything. If we are honest with ourselves, we know that these times will come when we least expect them. The plan does not need to be complicated. It could be simply, having a friend or family member care for our loved for a period. Extending their time at day care is also a temporary option. What ever we choose, we need to contact the people in our plan ahead of time, so that they can be ready on short notice.

I will make a plan, and be ready when an emergency presents itself.

Defining Who We Are

We can become consumed by our caregiving and can loose sight of who we really are. We struggle with the day-to-day demands, and somewhere along the way we realize that we have lost our identity. We have let the role of caregiver define who we are. We know that caregiving is a journey, and that it can be difficult when traveled alone; however, we also know we do not have to travel it alone. There are people waiting to help, if we just ask them. We cannot let our caregiving define who we are because we are so much more. We are parents, friends, lovers, grandparents with special attributes only we posses. It all comes down to looking at the big picture. We have and will accomplish many things along the caregiver road, and we must never lose sight of that. We also need to remember we are individuals first and caregivers second.

I will not let caregiving define who I am, and I will never lose sight of the beautiful person I am.

Prioritizing

During stressful times, our ability to think clearly diminishes and we lose the ability to prioritize. Being able to prioritize is a skill that will help us, especially when we are overwhelmed. We can start by taking time to figure out what are our priorities for today. When possible we need to stick to only things we can do today. "Tomorrow is another day Scarlet". It is the one day at a time philosophy. If there is something that we do not have to do today, it may be a wise decision to wait until tomorrow or even the next day. If it is that important it will still be there waiting for us tomorrow. Unforeseen thing are going to happen and that is OK. This is not a perfect world. By putting our activities in order of importance, we can establish a better daily routine. By doing daily planning, we will feel a sense of accomplishment.

I will prioritize the things I need to do and take one day at a time.

Faith above All

As caregivers we sometimes drift in and out of our faith, and our spiritual journey gets side tracked. Nevertheless, whatever path we take in our journey, we must continue to trust in our higher power. God is always present even when we think He has forsaken us. Our problems can seem overwhelming at times, and we feel alone and lost. Like the unconditional love we have for our loved one, we need to have unconditional trust in our higher power. Our faith is our hope. We must continually work on our spiritual well-being. We are, quite naturally, impatient in everything we do, but God is our source of patience. Sometimes we find it difficult to slow down long enough to hear God's answer to our prayers. God is with us every step of the way. He comforts our spirit and soothes our aching heart. We should never give up on him because He will not give up on us.

I will nurture my spiritual being and not give up my faith.

Travel

We have many avenues available to us if we want to travel, especially if our loved one is in the early stages. If we plan to take a trip and our loved one is going with us, we need to make some plans, so that our trip is as safe and stress free as possible. First, we must realize that their behavior may change because we are taking them out of their normal routine. The next thing we must consider is safety. Wandering can be a problem because they are in an unfamiliar place. Before we leave, we need to make sure they have an identification bracelet. It would also be a good idea to have some other form of identification sewn in their clothes or tucked in their wallet. We need to be vigilant about locking doors and making sure their new surroundings are safe. Their safety is our priority.

I will prepare a plan for traveling with my loved one so that our trip will be as safe as possible.

November 8

Redefining our Life

Redefining our life after the death of our loved one is difficult. During our caregiver days we felt guilty because we did not always trust our judgment; now we feel guilty because we could not make them better. We may even feel bad because we want to move on with our life. We have periods where we feel lonely and empty, and as uncomfortable as these feeling are, we want to get on with it. Our emotions feel unbalanced, and we are not sure what we want. There is something called the "one year rule." Very simply stated, it tells us to wait one year before we make any life altering decisions. We may also feel pressure from our friends or relatives to move to a different place, or make a big change in our life. Their suggestions are well intended, but in the end we must weigh the situation and make our own decisions. It is important that we do not rush these life-changing decisions.

I will make my decisions based on my needs and not on what others think I need.

The Quiet Place

We all have a quiet place within us. This is a place we go to gather our thoughts. We go there looking for solutions when we are having problems. We also go there, to talk to God and ask for help. When we retreat to this quiet place, we can open our minds and center our thoughts. This is a place where we feel at peace and can let go of anxiety and fear. Because our minds are filled with continual thoughts, it may take practice to get to this quiet state of mind. The pay-off is a sense of renewal and calmness that will help us face whatever problems we are faced with. When we quiet our mind, we have the opportunity to refocus. We can change our troubling thoughts to constructive attitudes. Deepak Chopra writes, "In stillness, inner energies spontaneously wake up and bring about the appropriate transformation for every situation."

I will search for my quiet inner place and begin to take retreat there when I feel stressed or confused.

Self -Talk

Self–talk refers to the dialogue that goes on inside our head when we are faced with conflict or challenges. The problem with self-talk is that it is usually negative. Overly critical thoughts cause us to beat ourselves up and make us feel miserable. "What was I thinking, how could I be so bad". These critical thoughts can be difficult to deal with, but the good news is, they can be managed. We can be the masters of our thoughts. If we get in touch with how we feel when we have these critical thoughts, we have taken the first step in ridding ourselves of them. The mere fact that they make us feel uncomfortable may be a good reason to change them. Our mind does not know the difference between what has actually happened, and what we have imagined has happened. Like gold medal winners, we can use visualization to make our minds think positively, and we can all be winners.

I will use my inner dialogue to think positively and make myself a winner.

Resources

The time to look for resources is before we need them. In a perfect world that is what would happen, but when we hear the final diagnosis that is the furthest from our minds. We may feel angry, sad and have an accumulation of emotions. Now time is more precious than ever. Our window of opportunity to find resources and make legal decisions is short. If we procrastinate in this area, our life as a caregiver will be chaotic and more stressful than necessary. We need to plan and find all the resources available so that when it is time to make decisions about finances or legal issues we know where to go and who to ask in. Advance planning allows us the time to think through our problems. It gives us control over our situation while relieving some of the burden. Yes, it is true, being the vigilant caregivers we are, we need to be in control.

I will examine all my resources so that I will be prepared to make informed decisions.

Flexibility

If there was ever a time to be flexible, it is now. Our loved one's abilities to do simple tasks, is declining. They move slower, their thought process is interrupted, and they do not always make good choices. Even with these restrictions we should let them do as much for themselves as possible. It does not really matter if their clothes do not match or that they will not let you shave them. No one ever died from not shaving or from wearing mismatched clothes. Our routines can no longer be the neat well-oiled routines they were before this disease. Schedules are things of the past. If a certain approach does not work, we may have to tap into our creativity and try something else. If we can remember to be patient, flexible and creative in our routines, we will be less frustrated. We need to adapt to the circumstances.

I will be flexible and adapt to my changing circumstances.

The Elephant

We all know about the elephant in the room. We know he is there, but we do not want to talk about it. We squeeze by it with niceties and talk of other things. We do not want to talk about the elephant in the room for fear of being hurt, or hurting someone else. There are issues and events that we refuse to acknowledge. We feel that if we ignore them they will go away. One such elephant may be the way we feel about our loved one's illness. If we are going to work through these feelings, we must acknowledge them and talk about them with someone so that we can rid ourselves of any guilt or fears that we have. We thought that what we were doing was a good coping mechanism, when, in fact, it was denial of what is happening in our life and that of our loved one.

I will acknowledge the elephant and learn to talk about my feelings and fears.

November 14

Imagination

Children can lie on the grass, look up at the fluffy clouds and imagine themselves to be animals or things. It did not matter that others could not visualize the shape, because children can and it brings them joy. These are precious moment of our childhood, and yet somehow, we have left them behind. As a child our minds were not so cluttered, and we had time to nurture our imagination. Now we rush through our hectic days too busy being grown ups. We forget how to dream and connect with the fun loving, carefree child within us. As adults we can benefit greatly by rediscovering some of that imaginative power. Harnessing the power of our imagination can have a positive impact on our lives. Sometimes we need to let go and just have fun. Muhammad Ali said, "The man who has no imagination has no wings."

I will rediscover my imagination and dream
of things that will bring me joy.

Hope

Giving up hope and just going through the motions of life putting one foot in front of the other is not enough. There is a difference between living and existing. When we just exist, we put ourselves in the survival mode and become isolated. When we give up hope, we miss the endless possibilities of our lives. Hope can be a wonderful thing that lets us see ourselves and our lives as unique. Hope is a quiet optimism. We know that however difficult our situation is, this too will pass. We do not have to surrender hope; we just need to change what we hope for. Hope is a gift we can give ourselves. When we hope, we have positive visions of what can be. Hope can be the "wind beneath our wings."

*I will look at life optimistically and give
myself the gift of hope.*

Worry

Worry can be a cycle. It can consume us, thus overwhelming us with anxiety. If we are in a constant state of worry, we can never find peace of mind. Nighttime and quiet moments can be the enemy if we are constant worriers. What a shame to waste these special moments. The monster in the closet is bigger and fiercer at night. We cannot stop worrying completely, but we can control what and when we worry. Worry is good in the "fight-or- flight" mode but how often do we meet a bear in our living room? Worrying is a habit that we have practiced for most of our adult life. We have been conditioned to worry. If we look back, did worry ever solve a problem for us? The answer is 100% no. It just holds us back and does not let us move forward. Worry is time wasted.

*I will not be consumed by worry or let
it waste my valuable time.*

Boundaries

We set our own personal boundaries, and it is up to us to let people know what they are. Our boundaries let people know what they can and cannot say or do to us. It's a type of filtering mechanism that sorts out things that make us and our loved one feel comfortable. We need to know what our boundaries are and how to enforce them. We also need to be assertive but not offensive when letting others know what our boundaries are. If someone is treating our loved one or us badly, it is our duty to let them know that their behavior is not acceptable to us. Once we have set our boundaries, there is no need to defend, debate, or explain them. When people cross our boundaries and we fail to say anything, we are giving our power and values away. These are the lines we draw that define our values. In essence, we teach people how to treat us.

*I will set personal boundaries and let people
know how I expect to be treated.*

Free Time

Yearning for free time to do what we want is almost an adult pastime. We look at free time to do what we want, as unattainable. Is it the lack of time that is the problem or is it the lack of motivation to create the time? Time management sounds so staunch, but if we look at it as making a plan and following it through, it becomes more palatable and attainable. Free time does not have to be measured in increments of hours. Some of our greatest pleasures can be found in moments. Smelling freshly brewed coffee, seeing the first robin of spring, watching the trees burst with color in autumn, can delight our senses. We need to take breaks to enjoy the simple things in life. Looking for free time in only large blocks will rob us of these sweet cherished moments. "When we are doing what we love, we don't care about time. For at least that moment, time does not exist and we are truly free." Marcia Wieder.

I will take time to refresh and enjoy
the small pleasures of life.

Emergencies

When emergencies arrive in our daily lives, they catch us off guard. So how can we prepare for an emergency if we are not expecting it? First, we must think of what would constitute an emergency in our lives. Having to go to the hospital in the middle of the night, or someone becoming very ill or dying are all types of emergencies that require fast action. We can prepare for some of these situations ahead of time. If we have all our medical papers, cards, and list of medications in one place, we should be able to access them immediately. Also keeping a list of emergency contacts and other pertinent information along with them is a good idea. We need to let friends and neighbors know where our emergency information is, as they are part of our personal support system. Being prepared for emergencies is crucial.

I will not be caught off guard in case of an emergency. I will make a plan and share it with my support system.

Forgetting

We get up and go into another room to get something; only to realize that when we get there, we have forgotten what it is we wanted. Although this can be unnerving to us, that is only a fraction of what our loved one goes through all the time. They want something, but they do not know what it is and probably cannot express it. If we pause for a moment or two, we usually remember what it was we were looking for, but our loved one does not have that luxury. As frightening as it is to us when we forget something, imagine how it must make them feel. Many times, they know something is wrong, but they do not know what. They are fighting against the odds every day. This insight should help us to be more understanding and patient. No one forgets on purpose.

Knowing that their disease is stealing away their memory, I will calm their fears and be more understanding.

Cooking

We do not have the time to look through magazines or cook books for new recipes. We are lucky if at the end of the day we have the strength or energy to make a full healthy meal. We may try to compensate by having a T.V. dinner or just snacking on whatever we find in the refrigerator. Occasionally this is all right, but we need to tap into our creative side so that we can fix nutritious meals at least five days a week. Remember the crock-pot that is in the back of the cupboard? It is time to dig it out. One-pot meals can be nutritious and convenient. Using this type of cooking is especially nice because there are usually enough left over for more than one meal. We can ask our friends in our support group to bring their favorite recipe to the next meeting for a recipe exchange. It is a win, win situation for all involved.

*I will try some one-pot meals to help me eat
well and save time in my day.*

Have a God Day

"Have a good day." This phrase is overly used and not always sincere, and yet we hear it all the time. Have a good day has become a standard, friendly way to end an interaction. What constitutes a good day for us, and are we willing to pursue it? Do we have what it takes, or are we just going to sit back and wait for it to happen? Today has great value, because many of the decisions we make today will affect our future. Are we going to be that fearless caregiver who can stand up to what today brings? If so we need to remember: Yesterday is gone; tomorrow it could be too late and someday may never come. Today really is the first day of our lives, and we need to use it to its fullest. A good day is what we make it.

I will enjoy today and make way for tomorrow.

Cry

As caregivers we are seen as the strong person in the family. Crying is usually not part of our demeanor; in fact, we may view it as being weak. We are very good at comforting others. As for ourselves, we hold our feelings inside, and this is not healthy. In order for us to come to terms with our feelings, we need someone to talk to, a person who will listen, and not pass judgment on us. Sometimes a good cry is good for the body and the soul. It can take all those pent up feelings and virtually wash them away, or at least make us feel better for the moment. There are tears of joy and tears of sadness, both reflect our humanity. We should never be too proud to cry. This is best said by Poet John Vance Cheney "The soul would have no rainbow had the eyes no tears".

I will not suppress my tears. I will let them flow and create a rainbow in my soul.

Our Pets

Our pets offer us unconditional love. They also bring us laughter and can brighten our day. It is a fact that by stroking a cat or dog, we can lower our blood pressure. The benefits of having a pet far out weigh the time it takes to care for them. Our human friends can offer us the social support we need, but our pets offer us endless entertainment and hours of comfort. They bring a sense of calm and well-being into our life and the life of our loved one. They ask very little of us, yet give so much. They have a second sense that knows when we are sad or sick. They curl up next to us to say, "it is ok I am here for you." We should never under estimate the power of our furry friends. It is said that when you die, you will know you are in heaven when all your pets come to greet you.

I will look at the benefits of having a pet and consider if it will work in my life.

Cycle of Guilt

What is guilt? Guilt is our feelings about our personal failures to live up to our self-imposed standards. It becomes a vicious circle of regrets and chips away at our self-esteem. It is totally self imposed. Nobody can make us feel guilty unless we let him or her. The danger of guilt is that it can cause us to become over responsive. We worry about everything we do and become over sensitive to other's needs. We give too much of ourselves, and are willing to do anything in an attempt to make everyone happy. Decisions become a matter of just right or wrong. We have no middle ground. We never let our guard down and are hyper-vigilant. Guilt can over power us if we do not stop and take control. If we are to overcome guilt, we need to forgive ourselves first and accept who we are. Loving caring human beings.

*I will deal with my guilt and forgive myself
so that I can move forward.*

Thanksgiving

Despite the trials and tribulations of being a caregiver on this day, we have much to be thankful for. Caregiving has given us physical, mental and spiritual abilities that have strengthened us. We have learned how to be patient and how to laugh, even when the going gets tough. We have found the courage to try new things. We can now look at the big picture and anticipate our loved one's needs. Our sensitivity has been heightened as we learn to come to terms with our emotions. All of these things have groomed us to be the best caregiver we can be. We can give thanks using the words of Ralph Waldo Emerson, "For each new morning with its light, for rest and shelter of the night, for health and food, for love and friends, for everything Thy goodness sends. We give thanks."

I will give thanks for all that I have and all that I am.

Gratitude

Our attitude controls how we see the world and how we relate to it. In his book <u>Attitudes of Gratitude</u> author M.J. Ryan, teaches us how an attitude of gratitude inspires us to think positively and live a more joyous life. It is hard sometimes to feel grateful when we are tired and lonely. What is there to feel grateful about anyway? Could it possibly be as simple as we have food on our table and a roof over our head? The answer is yes, and that is just the beginning. Gratitude turns what we have into enough, and more. Even in the midst of extremely trying circumstances, we can usually find something for which we can be truly grateful. By being conscious of what we have and not what we do not have, we will feel gratitude and it will show in our attitude. One of the best things about an attitude of gratitude is that it is contagious.

I will improve my attitude and make it one of gratitude.

November 28

Home

"I want to go home." People with Alzheimer's echo this familiar phrase a thousand times a day. Even though they have lived in the same home for 20 or 30 years, they do not see it as their home now. Their body is not where their mind is at these moments. What they are probably looking for is the home of their childhood, or it may be that they want to see a loved one who has long passed. Not finding comfort in the place where you live is sad indeed. So here, we go again telling them a therapeutic fib: "I'll take you home right after we have dinner." To use reality therapy would be cruel. Recognizing their feelings of insecurity and validating them will usually solve the problem temporarily. If nothing else, it will calm them for a moment, giving us a little time to regroup ourselves mentally.

I will validate my loved one. When they ask to go home, I will calmly redirect and comfort them.

Bitterness

Anger and focusing on what is wrong can suck our energy, and we will become bitter people where nothing seems right. Bitterness can breed resentment and makes us develop a critical attitude. These are not admirable traits. People do not want to be around someone that is constantly bitter about their plight in life. Of course there are things in our life that make us sad and angry, but that doesn't' mean we can cling to them forever. A favorite saying often expressed today is "just get over it," and maybe that's exactly what we need to do. It does not mean we cannot feel sad when bad thing happen. We just cannot continue to hold on to negative thoughts forever, and play poor me. People do not want to be with "poor me." Who wants to be with a person that makes them feel bad? Life is too short to be bitter.

I have no place for bitterness; life is to short.

Journey of Caregiving

The journey of caregiving is like no other. Unlike a vacation, we do not get to plan ahead of time. Even when a family is going to have a baby, there are books to read and nine months to prepare. They even get a party and everyone gives gifts to help in this new role of life. When we become caregivers, no one will throw us a party. We have made our decision. We are determined to take this journey even though we find ourselves filled with self-doubt. From the very beginning we need to have a realistic view of the situation so that we can be familiar with the options that are available to us. We may struggle with our emotions and find it hard at first, but we have resolved to accept this challenge. We will work through the new challenges and demands and lay the groundwork of loving care. We will ask God for guidance in all that we do.

I will move through my caregiving journey with grace so that in the end I can say, "Well Done."

December

∾

*"My idea of Christmas, whether old-fashioned
or modern, is very simple: loving others. Come
to think of it, why do we have to wait for
Christmas to do that?"*

Bob Hope

Holidays

The holidays are traditional times where we gather together with our family and friends, or at least we did in the past. Unfortunately, holidays can be difficult times because we feel additional pressure. We can feel overwhelmed in an effort to maintain our holiday traditions. Although we need to be somewhat flexible, we also need to maintain our normal routine as much as possible. This will help in the continuity of care for our loved one. We know what is best for them and we can set the pace. If we are going to enjoy the holidays, we need to communicate. This is not a time to feel guilty. We know our limitations and our family and friends need to understand our situation, but this will not be possible unless we tell them how things are. By setting the boundaries, we can now enjoy the holidays on our terms.

I will set the boundaries when celebrating with my family so my loved one and I can continue to enjoy the holidays.

Driving Intervention

One of the most difficult decisions we have to make as caregivers to loved ones with dementia is when to intervene and stop them from driving. Some caregivers will act as a co-pilot and give directions and instructions as to when to stop or go. We should not be afraid of them getting lost as much as we should fear their slow reaction time and distance perception. Their ability to process information makes them a danger to themselves and others. It all comes down to this would we rather have them mad at us, or let them get into an accident that could costs lives? Physicians are mandated to report medical conditions that would impair driving. This may be the good time to have a candid discussion with their doctor so that he can help intervene.

I will begin to evaluate my loved one's driving ability and be honest with myself about their driving capability.

Social Isolation

Social isolation puts us at risk for physical and mental deterioration. Because of our loved one's disease we slowly enter into an isolated state. Our friends may stop calling or stopping by. We do not go out in public with our loved one because it is embarrassing, or just too much work to get them ready. Each time we fall prey to these moments, we relinquish our personal need for social contact. The results of isolation are many. Loneliness, burnout, stress and personal health issues. Knowing that we are at risk for isolation, we should begin early to take charge of our daily lives. Recognizing the resources that are available to us and using them is a good first step. Sharing our daily lives with our friends and family will allow them the opportunity to help and share the burden. Isolation does not have to make us its prisoner.

I will avoid isolation and take charge of my life.

Aging is not a Disease

We sometimes feel like aging is a bad thing. Our culture is not always kind when looking at the aging population. People often think that Alzheimer's is a normal part of aging. They come to believe that an older person is falling apart mentally and physically. They get confused and have a hard time deciphering slowing down, from disability. Just because a person is older doesn't mean that they are impaired, or somehow disabled. Although the risk of disease and disability increase with advancing age, poor health is not an inevitable part of aging. We need to dispel these myths. We are as old as we think we are. There are many young 70, 80, and 90 year olds. They are active, alert, and enjoying life. We, as aging caregivers, can run circles around our younger counterparts. Aging is not a disease. So how old would we be if we did not know how old we are?

I am only as old as I feel, and I will work at keeping myself physically and mentally young

Perception of Life

Living a full life can be simple if we do not complicate it. We are given the privilege of living a full, meaningful life if we are willing to open ourselves to happiness. It is a natural state of being human, and this is evidenced by watching babies for a couple of minutes. They do not have a problem being happy, they just are. One of the tricks to being happy is to get into the habit of looking for the good things in our life. Spending time regretting what we do not have is a waste of time. Our life will have its ups and downs, its peaks and valleys, but how we perceive them makes the difference. Perception is the key. We need to do what we need to do, and be grateful for the opportunities life gives us. Peter Marshall hit it on the head when he said; "When we long for life without difficulties, remind us that oaks grow strong in contrary winds and diamonds are made under pressure."

I will take pleasure in my life and live it to its fullest.

December 6

Vacation

Although short respites are good, taking a real vacation is really necessary. We all need time to regroup and reflect. We also need time to interact with others outside of our care circle. Having something to look forward to can be very exciting. The old excuses such as, "no one can care for them like I can," or "what if something happens when I am not there" are no longer valid. The quality of care our loved one receives from us is proportionate to our personal health and well-being. It may be true that someone other than us cannot give the same care, but that does not mean the care is not good. As caregivers we need occasional freedom from everyday responsibilities. We do have a life of our own, and we need to recognize that. We deserve to have periods of time not devoted to caring for someone else, however much we love that person.

*Out of love and respect for my loved one and myself, I will
take some extended time alone.*

Pro-active

Pro-active caregivers look ahead and plan. Being proactive means thinking and acting ahead, and this means using foresight. Many things we need to do or find out in order to make a good plan are not always pleasant, but need to be done none the less. If we arm ourselves with the knowledge of what may lie ahead we are more able to cope with the difficult times that come in caregiving. We are the only ones who know what we are capable of; therefore our plan needs to fit our needs. Crises happen to everyone, but some can be prevented if we are pro-active. By being on top of our situations, we have a better chance of resolving and accepting the changes that come with the disease process. As pro-active caregivers, we may not always know what lies ahead, but we do know we will be ready when it happens.

I will take a pro-active approach to my caregiving.

Natural Feelings

It is normal to feel some relief when our loved one passes on. We have watched them suffer and slip away little by little each day. However, our feelings of relief can also make us feel guilty. This is by no means a reflection of not loving enough, or not caring enough. It is a reflection of the fact that we are human beings who have reached the end of our emotional rope, and we are afraid that we may not be able meet the challenges ahead. We have suffered and feel alone and exhausted. We may also feel angry because things are now out of our control. Not being able to communicate with them in the later stages of the disease is distressing. We have suffered anticipatory grief for years, and the end has finally come. We have cared for them according to their wishes, and our unconditional love will never die.

I will love and care for my loved one until the end, and when that time comes, I will not look back with regret.

Tradition

Traditions are a direct reflection of our family beliefs and values. They connect us to people, places and time. Traditions are more than routines, which are ordinary everyday activities. Traditions give us comfort and show our love for each other. Because of the many dimensions of caregiving it may become more difficult to personally perform these customs. When this happens, it is time to pass the baton. The word tradition comes from the Latin word tradio, which means to hand down. Keeping traditions alive is what make us unique and creates a family bond. Traditions can give us a sense of timelessness and span generations. Traditions are not just for the holidays. Our lives are interlaced with them, from making a favorite family recipe to reciting a family prayer. Traditions are not traditions unless they are passed on. "Tradition is everything," said the fiddler. Now is the time to pass them on.

I will pass down our family traditions so that they can remain part of my family's lives.

Choices

Is there a right time to make the decision when to place our loved one in a facility? First, this is a personal decision. No two person's breaking points or circumstances are the same. What we need to look at are safety issues, hygiene, nutrition, and of course, behavior. We also need to look at our own health. We all know that caregiving can be overwhelming at best. We should not look at placement as a sign that we have failed, and our guilt has to give way to practicality. It is best if it can be a family decision, but again that is not always possible. Most of all we need to stay away from the guilt trip. Guilt and feelings of failure will only cloud our judgment. When our loved one enters a nursing home, our caregiving duties are far from over. We will always need to be there to advocate for them.

I will still my guilt and give way to practicality, when it becomes necessary for extended care of my loved one.

One Pharmacy

Medicines that are strong enough to help us can also be strong enough to hurt us. We need to get to know our pharmacist and make them a part of our health care team. We should try to have all our prescriptions filled at the same pharmacy. The more we work in a trio-us, our doctor and our pharmacist-the more we will benefit from our medications. Our pharmacist can tell us how and when to take our medicine, whether a drug may interact with or affect another medicine or whether there can be any side effects. It is also a good idea to have our pharmacist check our over the counter drugs. Misuse of medication can cause illness or worse death. Our pharmacist can keep track of all our medications and will be able to tell us if a new drug might cause problems. Overall, it is a good idea to have all our medication records in one place. We need to be smart consumers when it comes to medication.

I will us one pharmacy and make my pharmacist part of my health care team.

Children

Children and adolescents can be strongly affected when a loved family member is stricken with Alzheimer's. If the loved one is close to them, they can feel sad, helpless, and even embarrassed. We need to deal with them gently, because this is a time in their life when they are growing and maturing. We first need to be open with them and not overwhelm them with too much information. If you can get the dialogue started, it is important to listen carefully and let them ask questions. Giving them this information will help them deal with the changes, especially those of inappropriate behavior. Above all, we should not judge them. Remember, this is a family disease and adults have a difficult time talking openly about it. We are only human and do not have all the answers. The main thing is that we reassure them that we are ok; we love them and understand what they are feeling.

*I will speak to the children in a straightforward
and empathetic manner.*

Love of Self

There are times when we feel that no one loves us or cares about what we are going through. These feelings are normal, and they happen to most caregivers. When these feeling present themselves, we need to tap into our inner love of self. Self-love can be a powerful force. It is a conscious awareness of who we are. Loving ourselves is not the same as being selfish or being a narcissist. We are warm nurturing people who have taken on a job that is shunned by many. We posses extraordinary skills and compassion. We accept who we are, but continue to strive to be the best that we can. Loving our selves also means taking care of our bodies, minds, and spirits. When we love ourselves, we automatically attract people who see those qualities in us. In life, positive energy attracts positive people and things. That is the power of self-love.

I will practice self-love and take care of
my body, mind, and soul.

Spirit of Giving

The spirit of giving has two components, one is the giver and the other the receiver. As caregivers we often feel more comfortable in giving rather than receiving. It is in our nature. When our children were growing up, we gave all we could to them, even though it meant sacrificing for ourselves. We appear to others to be strong and in total control. We put up a good front so that others will not see our suffering. We act as if nothing is wrong and then we wonder why others are not sympathizing with us. People cannot help what they do not see. Our egos get in the way. We want to be seen as strong, and at the same time, we want help. Our actions contradict our needs. Being a martyr benefits no one. One of the greatest gifts we can give ourselves is to learn how to ask and receive help.

*I will keep control of my life and learn
how to receive as well as give.*

Long Term Pain-Short Term Pain

Our goal in life is not to live where there are no challenges, but rather to be able to live through those challenges. All of us in some way have to deal with difficulty and challenge. Our life is a series of challenges. We can choose to meet them head on or let them overwhelm us. The challenges in our life allow us to see ourselves at our best and our worst. How we deal with our challenges determines how we experience life. We can see it as a struggle or as an adventure. There is long-term pain and short-term pain. If we try to avoid the challenge, that is long-term pain and nothing will be resolved. If we meet it head-on with forethought and confidence, will be able to conquer the challenge. Challenge can only be overcome when we acknowledge it and then move through it. The decision is ours.

*I will move through my challenges and use
the avenue of short-term pain.*

December 16

Expectations

Unrealistic expectations of our loved one or of ourselves, can lead to stress and anxiety. We know what we are capable of, and yet we continue to try to do things that we are unable to do. Our loved one is losing the ability to reason and can no longer work a problem through but sometimes we think they are being obstinate on purpose. We need to consider their limitations when we want them to perform a task or answer a question. Expectations are the key to developing an effective care strategy, but this disease throws us a curve ball because it is progressive, continually changing our challenges. What worked today may not work tomorrow. If we set the bar too high and do not consider these limitations, we are inviting problems. We need to try our best, and that is good enough.

I will keep my expectations realistic and do my best in all that I do.

The Ripple Effect

Even our most inconsequential actions can have a butterfly effect. The butterfly theory states that if a butterfly chances to flap his wings in Beijing in March, then by August, hurricane patterns in the Atlantic will be completely different. Every thing we do, everything we have learned eventually is put into action. This action affects more people than we know. We have learned how to make bathing more comfortable for our loved one. We have made them feel safe and happy. We take this experience to our support meeting and share it. Others try it, and their loved one feels better, and on and on. The people we help in our every day lives can never be measured. Everything we do and do not do has an effect on someone. Each choice we make, each action we take, causes a ripple effect.

I will carefully choose my actions, as they may become the actions of others.

December 18

Fear

Fear is a common problem from which none of us is immune. There are some good types of fear, like fearing to walk on thin ice, but the fears that usually consume us are the unhealthy fears. They can generate from past experiences, or they can be the fear of the unknown. As a caregiver we may fear that we are not doing the right things. We are fearful that the future is going to be bad no matter what we do. One of the biggest fears is what will happen to our loved one if something bad happens to us. Although these are legitimate fears, we should not let them consume our every thought; if we do, they will take control of our lives, and we will not be able to move forward. We need to confront our fears so that we gain back control over our daily lives.

Today I will confront my fears and gain
back control of my life.

Incontinence

Incontinence is the involuntary loss of bladder or bowel control. Incontinence can be upsetting and humiliating for the person with dementia, and stressful for us as caregivers. Our approach to this problem will make a great deal of difference to the outcome. If we see it as disgusting or something they are doing on purpose, we are heading for a long road of grief. If we have had their health checked and the incontinence is not medical, then we need to address their needs. There is a lot of information on how to deal with incontinence, but in the end, we must do what works best for us. They and we may find this hard to accept because it is such an intimate part of life. We need to be conscious of what we call the incontinence garments. No adult wants to hear the word diaper. Since we never really know how much our loved one understands, we need to choose our words carefully and approach the changing task as lovingly as possible.

*I will use a gentle approach in dealing with
my loved one's incontinence.*

December 20

Quality Verse Quantity

When we look at the quality of our life, it is not how much we live, have, or do, but what we make of each moment that counts. When we speak about quality of life, we are talking about the degree of well being, comfort, and happiness we feel in these moments. Often in the pursuit of quantity, we cheat ourselves of quality. If we love chocolate but are forced to eat it all day, every day, we would soon tire of it. Could that be possible? We need to put into perspective just what is satisfying about our life. Everyone is working towards something, so what is it that makes us happy now? If we take the time to focus on what makes us happy, we may be surprised at how little it really takes to make us feel content. Being happy does not mean that things are perfect; it means that we resolve to look beyond life's imperfections.

I will look past the imperfections of life and focus on what makes me happy now.

The Enemy

"We have met the enemy and he is us" is a line from the long-running daily comic strip "Pogo" by Walt Kelly. Was he looking in our window? No, but we know that many times we are our own worst enemy. We try too hard to meet our unrealistic expectations. When we do not meet them, we become angry with ourselves. Anger is caused when something, someone, or we fail to meet our expectations. We will never win the battle or beat the enemy if we set goals that are unobtainable or to difficult too accomplish. When we expect too much, we are in constant motion; we feel that we are never done, or that we could do it better. To beat the enemy we must recognize him and come to terms with what this battle is costing us.

I will stop being my own worst enemy and
keep my expectations realistic.

December 22

Choose Wisely

Not everything is worth fighting over. We need to pick and choose our battles wisely. If we make our decision based on what is right not who is right, we have the opportunity to sort out the importance of the issues. No one is always right, and it is not about winning any way. It is about doing the right thing at the right time. We need to save our energy for the things that are important. If we look at every issue as a battle, we become negative and that is a waste of precious time. When we take a moment to step back and examine the issue, we may see it in a different light. It may not be as important as we first thought. Once we recognize what is important, we can then let go of what is not.

I will base my decisions on what is right, not who is right.

Acknowledging the Holidays

It may have started with not putting up the Christmas tree or not setting up the Menorah or the candles for Quanza. Our holiday memory from before our loved one developed Alzheimer's has darkened what usually is a joyful season. Things may have gotten so bad that we dread the arrival of the holidays. Instead of dreading them, we need to find less stressful ways to celebrate them. We can start by making adjustments and considerations to improve our chance for a happy holiday. We need to acknowledge these holiday even though we are in a difficult situation. We can start by asking ourselves what would be the least stressful and meaningful way to celebrate the season. We should not let our role as a caregiver diminish our celebration or overshadow the simple pleasure of being with family and friends. The holidays are days to be remembered and cherished for years to come, and we do not have to give them up.

I will look for less stressful ways to celebrate the holidays with my family and friends.

Aging Gracefully

We can approach our aging in one of two ways. The first approach is aging gracefully. The second is to approach it kicking and screaming. Aging gracefully does not mean giving up. If we move toward it kicking and screaming, we may miss the many lessons it has taught us. It is not easy to age gracefully in our youth worshiping society. Throughout the ages, people have been searching for the elusive "Fountain of Youth." Aging is not a bad thing, infact the alternative is really bad. If we look at what we have gained from past experiences of our life rather than what we have lost, we will be able to move gracefuly into the land of wisdom and knowledge called aging. There are no creams or magic pills that can give us the wisdom that aging can. "Aging is not 'lost youth' but a new stage of opportunity and strength." Betty Friedan.

I will look toward aging with an opened mind and move towards it gracefully.

Honoring Ourselves

Today we need to take the time to honor ourselves. We need to acknowledge our strengths, our wisdom, and creativity. Honoring ourselves means, we recognize our needs and the right to fulfill them. We need to stop taking ourselves so seriously. Very few things are as serious as we think they are. By honoring ourselves, we become more conscious of our needs and become as available to ourselves as we are to others. There is much good in us, and we need to take the time to recognize and celebrate the loving, caring person we are. So often, we focus so much on our flaws and the things that we have done wrong, that we cannot see the good in ourselves. Self-honoring raises our self-esteem level and renders us more content. If we do not recognize and honor ourselves, we cannot expect others to do so. By honoring our body, we honor our soul.

Today I will honor myself and say, "Job well done."

Goals

What is our main goal on our caregiving journey? Certainly, it is not to cure our loved one of this disease, because we know it just will not happen. No one gets out of this disease alive. We must now adapt to the condition rather than the cure. As harsh as this sounds it does not mean that we have to give up our quality of life. We can still experience tender moments, happiness and joy; in fact, we will be more aware of these special times and take pleasure in them. Life as we know it is not over, only the circumstances have changed. If we are realistic about what we want to achieve, the outcome is more than attainable. Our main goal should be to improve the quality of life for our loved one. We will never catch a fish unless we put our line in the water.

*I will set realistic goals and strive to improve
my loved one's quality of life.*

Empowerment

Empowerment is an overused buzzword in our society today, but if we are going to rise above our daily challenges, we need to feel empowered. When we are empowered, we are more open to learning new things and finding needed resources. It fosters the "can do" attitude and gives us the power and energy to get things done. When we are empowered, we feel confident in our ability to make decisions and do what is best for our loved one. Empowerment can be a kind of personal power where we feel secure in who and what we are. We can handle adversity with grace and have control over our destiny. We have a positive impact on what is happening to and around us. When we harness the power within us, we will achieve the quality of life we deserve. Our life has a sense of harmony.

My personal power allows me to feel secure in
who I am; I will respect it.

December 28

Inspiration

When we grow up, we sometimes forget to dream. Maybe the reason is that we get too busy or consumed with our pressing demands. We place limits on ourselves that block inspiration from coming through. Inspiration comes in many ways and forms. It is all around us, but we can only see it if our minds are open. Inspiration can be found in magazines, in talking with others, or just reading a word that jogs our creativity memory. Inspiration usually comes to us at quiet times, when our minds are not cluttered, and we give ourselves permission to reflect on new thoughts or ideas. Inspiration is a magical thing. It can motivate us to try new ways of doing everyday things. This Zen Proverb explains it well: "When the student is ready, the teacher will appear."

I will keep an open mind so that inspiration
can find its place in my life.

Winners

We are all winners. Much like children playing T ball, there are no losers. We cannot control the hand we were dealt, but we can control how we play it. Although this disease has placed many burdens on us and asked us to do things we never thought possible, we accomplished them. We learned to balance hope with realism. Our family role may have changed, but our love has not. We have learned new things and helped others on their journey. We have practiced tough love and patience at the same time. We have have had moments of joy and moments of heartache. Our patience has been tried but we have come out strengthened. When all is said and done, we have embraced the challenge. We are masters of what we do. We are all Winners.

I will adopt a winning attitude and use the law of attraction to attract other winners.

December 30

Wonderful Life

In the movie <u>It's a Wonderful Life</u> an angel named Clarence shows the main character George how much his life means by showing him how the world would be without him. This Christmas classic can give us thought as to what our loved one's life would be with out us. We sometimes fail to recognize the full extent and affect our caregiving makes. Routine things such as bathing, eating, and seemingly everyday tasks would not be done with out us. The care and guidance that we give are not measurable. We have the opportunity during this holiday season to look at our life and all that we have to offer. We need to take pride in all that we do. This is not a job for the faint of heart. It takes exceptional fortitude and love to carry out our mission. We care with all our heart and soul, and our heroic efforts are making a tremendous difference in the lives of our loved ones and others.

I will continue to make a difference in my loved one's life and give thanks for the opportunity to do so.

p_{in}

Caregiving is like dancing on the head of a pin. We do not have to be the best dancer we just need to keep our balance. We dance to the music of days gone by. We swing with the gratitude that God has given us this time to be together. We are proud of our accomplishments and look forward to whatever challenges lie ahead. Our love grows stronger, and our commitment is forever. We delight in the knowledge that guides us through this journey. Life can be complicated...or not. The choice is really ours. We have the courage and stamina to keep the delicate balance that defines us as caregivers extraordinaire.

May you be blessed in all that you do.

Index:

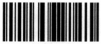

1771968

Made in the USA